the Electronic Health Record

for the PHYSICIAN'S OFFICE

with  for the medical office

Amy M. DeVore, MSTD, CPC, CMA (AAMA)

Program Director
Practicum Coordinator
Assistant Professor
Medical Assisting Program
Butler County Community College
Butler, Pennsylvania

ELSEVIER

3251 Riverport Lane
St. Louis, Missouri 63043

The Electronic Health Record for the Physician's Office with
SimChart for the Medical Office   ISBN: 978-0-323-44731-7

Notices

Knowledge and best practice in this field are constantly changing. As new research and experience
broaden our understanding, changes in research methods, professional practices, or medical treatment may become necessary.

Practitioners and researchers must always rely on their own experience and knowledge in evalu-
ating and using any information, methods, compounds, or experiments described herein. In using
such information or methods they should be mindful of their own safety and the safety of others,
including parties for whom they have a professional responsibility.

With respect to any drug or pharmaceutical products identified, readers are advised to check the
most current information provided (i) on procedures featured or (ii) by the manufacturer of each
product to be administered, to verify the recommended dose or formula, the method and duration
of administration, and contraindications. It is the responsibility of practitioners, relying on their
own experience and knowledge of their patients, to make diagnoses, to determine dosages and the
best treatment for each individual patient, and to take all appropriate safety precautions.

To the fullest extent of the law, neither the Publisher nor the authors, contributors, or editors,
assume any liability for any injury and/or damage to persons or property as a matter of products
liability, negligence or otherwise, or from any use or operation of any methods, products, instructions, or ideas contained in the material herein.

ISBN: 978-0-323-44731-7

Content Strategist: Jennifer Janson
Developmental Editor: Elizabeth Goldstein/Heather Rippetoe
Publishing Services Manager: Jeff Patterson
Project Manager: Jeanne Genz
Design Direction: Paula Catalano
Marketing Manager: Anne Simon

Printed in the United States of America

Last digit is the print number: 9 8 7 6 5 4 3 2 1

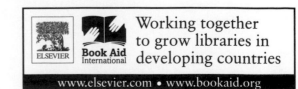

*To my Family— Roy, Carly, and Aden. I'm so proud of us. I appreciate
your support and patience while I follow my dreams.*

*To the amazing, supportive, and innovative SCMO development team:
John Dolan, Kate Gilliam, Kevin Korinek, and Julie Pepper.
It doesn't feel like work when you are doing something you enjoy.
You have all helped to make that a reality to me.*

In memory of Susan Cole. Thanks for giving me a chance.

Preface

As an instructor I started writing this book to fulfill a need for my classroom. My students were going into externships and employment ill-prepared for the electronic office. Current accreditation requirements are changing the way instructors teach medical assisting. Students are gaining employment in electronic, paper-based, and hybrid offices. How does an instructor properly prepare students for the different environments they may be exposed to? This text prepares students for their first job using the electronic health record.

The purpose of *The Electronic Health Record for the Physician's Office* is to provide instructors a seamless instructional transition from paper-based records offices to electronic health records offices. This text is not just about technology but the application of technology in health care.

The approach includes both theory and hands-on work for the students. *The Electronic Health Record for the Physician's Office* focuses on both the electronic health record and the administrative procedures that use the EHR. The review questions offer critical thinking and problem solving for students. The EHR exercises keep students engaged by allowing them to simulate work in a real physician's office, helping them understand theory as they put what they learn to practice.

This textbook features the SimChart for the Medical Office, but its concepts are broad enough to cover most EHR software available to medical practices. Students who complete *The Electronic Health Record for the Physician's Office* should be able to transfer their knowledge to other EHR software. Although the screens may look different, the basic functions are the same. It is my hope that my textbook will offer students an advantage in the job market over others who have not had a detailed exposure to electronic health records. After completing the course using *The Electronic Health Record for the Physician's Office*, the student will feel prepared and confident working with an EHR.

The web-based software allows students to access the product from school and home. This is important for the changing instructional environment. This text can accommodate traditional classrooms as well as hybrid and online courses. The portability of the software allows students more practice, repetition, and exploration.

ORGANIZATION

The textbook is organized in a work-text format and designed to combine both theory and practice throughout each chapter. Common tasks and features of EHR software are explained one step at a time using examples and screenshots from SimChart for the Medical Office. EHR exercises then follow, allowing students a hands-on opportunity to apply the previously learned concepts.

DISTINCTIVE FEATURES

- *Trends and Applications* give students real-life examples of how EHR systems are being used to improve healthcare, and how they may be used in the future.
- *Easing the Transition* discusses common issues that often arise during the conversion from paper to electronic medical records. Students gain insight into the conversion process, a situation they may encounter during an externship or job.
- *Security Checkpoints* explore issues of EHR security and patient privacy. Attention is directed to issues of security and privacy as they pertain to EHR systems.
- *Critical Thinking Exercises* appear throughout each chapter and provide students with thought-provoking questions to enhance learning and stimulate discussion.

LEARNING AIDS

- Each chapter opens with a list of the newest national curriculum competencies for CAAHEP that are covered within the chapter.
- Well-developed *Learning Objectives* follow the organizational flow of each chapter. They are also summarized at the end of each chapter for student review.
- *Key Terms* are listed and defined in the beginning of each chapter and bolded where they appear in the text. The key terms are also available in a glossary at the back of the book for quick reference.
- EHR exercises are integrated throughout each chapter, providing students an opportunity to practice with actual software and reinforce key concepts. **Important note:** The EHR exercises increase in difficulty based on the knowledge gained, and some depend on the successful completion of previous exercises. Therefore, the EHR exercises should be completed in the order in which they appear in the text.

- A variety of *Chapter Review Activities* are available at the end of each chapter, allowing students to assess their knowledge of the material. Activities include key terms review, matching, true/false, and additional opportunities to practice with the software.

ANCILLARIES

Evolve Resources with TEACH Instructor Resources (TIR) provides students and instructors with supplemental features that complement this textbook. The website also allows students and instructors to stay current with trends, developments, and news of the electronic heath record.

For the Student

- Direct access to SimChart for the Medical Office.

For the Instructor

- Answer Keys provide answers to the *EHR Exercises*, *Critical Thinking Exercises*, and *Chapter Review Activities*.
- TEACH Instructor Resources for each chapter are available on the Evolve site, including:
- TEACH Lesson Plans provide instructors with customizable lesson plans for each chapter.
- PowerPoints provide instructors with talking points, thought-provoking questions, and unique ideas for lectures.
- ExamView testbank offers instructors test items for a wide variety of examination styles.

—Amy DeVore

Contents

chapter 1

Introduction to Electronic Health Records

Chapter Outline

Commission on Accreditation of Allied Health Education Programs (CAAHEP) Competencies

1. Discuss applications of electronic technology in effective communication.
2. Discuss principles of using electronic medical records (EMRs).
3. Execute data management using electronic healthcare records such as the EMR.
4. Use the Internet to access information related to the medical office.

Chapter Objectives

1. Explore the history and current use of patient health records, their importance to individuals' health, and their contribution to the healthcare system.
2. Become familiar with the content of a typical electronic health record (EHR).
3. Define *documentation*, and explain who documents in the medical record.
4. Discuss ownership of the health record.
5. List and explain the eight core functions of an EHR.
6. Describe the basic functions and advanced clinical decision support features of EHR software.
7. Define *practice management software*, and explain how it is used with the EHR system.
8. Describe advantages of EHR systems.
9. Describe disadvantages of EHR systems.
10. Discuss EHR adoption rates and who is using EHR systems.
11. Identify the roles of various healthcare professionals in implementing an EHR system.
12. Investigate various professional organizations aimed at promoting the use of EHR systems.

Key Terms

account ledger   An accounting billing document that lists services provided, copayments made by the patient, reimbursement received from the patient's insurance company, and outstanding amount owed.

audit   A review of employee activity within the EHR system, including an examination of which files were accessed or modified, when, and why.

Certification Commission for Healthcare Information Technology (CCHIT)   A recognized certification body for EHR systems and their networks. The CCHIT is an independent, voluntary private-sector initiative whose goal is to accelerate the adoption of health information technology.

chief complaint   The patient's stated primary reason for seeking treatment.

clinical decision support (CDS)   A set of patient-centered tools embedded within EHR software that can be used to improve patient safety, ensure that care conforms to published protocol for specific conditions, and reduce duplicate or unnecessary care and its associated costs.

computerized provider order entry (CPOE)   An EHR function that allows a physician or other prescriber to order medications and tests using an automated format; CPOE can reduce prescribing errors, delays, and duplication and simplify inventory and billing processes.

continuity of care   A key aspect of quality that encompasses planning and coordination of care, communication among members of the healthcare team, and accessibility and transportability of information.

copayment   A fixed sum of money that is paid by the patient, usually at the time medical services are rendered.

day sheet   A register for daily business transactions; also called a *day journal*.

documentation   The process of recording data about a patient's health history and status, including clinical observations and progress notes, diagnoses of illnesses and injuries, plans of care, patient education and self-care instructions given, vital signs taken, physical assessment findings, laboratory and imaging test results, medical treatments prescribed or administered, surgeries performed, and outcomes; the term can also refer to the chronologic record that results from such data entry.

electronic health record (EHR)   A computerized patient health record that allows the electronic management of a patient's health information by multiple healthcare providers and stores the patient's contact information, legal documents, demographic data, and administrative information; the term can also refer more broadly to a system that manages such records.

electronic transcription   Data entry into the EHR using handwriting recognition, voice recognition, electronic sentence building, scanning, and other means.

Key Terms—cont'd

encounter   A documented interaction or visit between a patient and healthcare provider.

interoperability   The ability of separate EHR systems to share information in compatible formats.

patient information form (PIF)   A form used to gather data about the patient, including basic demographic information, medical insurance data, and emergency contact.

practice management software (PMS)   Software used in a medical office to accomplish administrative (nonclinical) tasks, including entry of patient demographics, record-keeping for insurance and other billing transactions, appointment scheduling, and advanced accounting functions.

structured data entry   Documentation using controlled vocabulary via preloaded data, drop-down boxes, radio buttons, and sentence builders.

third-party payer   A party other than the patient, spouse, parent, or guardian who is responsible for paying all or part of the patient's medical costs, typically the insurance company.

WHAT IS A MEDICAL RECORD?

History of Medical Records

Nearly as long as there have been physicians, there have been medical records. A patient medical record is a complete physical collection of an individual's healthcare information. Chunyu Yi, who was born in China in approximately 200 BCE, is one of the first physicians known to have kept records on the patients he treated. His written observations of patient signs and symptoms are one of the first known forms of patient documentation. A hospital in Damascus, Syria, built in 706 CE, was perhaps among the first in history to adopt the widespread use of medical records.

Medical records and death ledgers were kept during the plagues that swept through Europe during the fourteenth and seventeenth centuries. In the United States during the Civil War era, soldiers' medical records documented "nervous disease" (later known as shell shock and now posttraumatic stress disorder), as well as injuries suffered in combat and infectious diseases contracted in the crowded, unsanitary military camps. Between 1892 and 1954, medical records were created for most of the 12 million immigrants who passed through Ellis Island, eager to begin their new lives in America. The record served as proof that the person had been deemed able-bodied and free of communicable diseases, such as tuberculosis and smallpox, which would have prompted quarantine or deportation.

Of course, medical records haven't always been used in the service of good ends. Nazi physicians often kept meticulous records on each "patient" forced to participate in their gruesome, cruel experiments. Between 1932 and 1972, researchers documented the signs, symptoms, and complications of syphilis in the records of hundreds of African-American men during the infamous Tuskegee syphilis experiment. The men were denied proper care and allowed to suffer long after penicillin was found to be a highly effective treatment for syphilis.

These researchers, fortunately, represent an exception to the generally high standard of conduct observed by members of the medical and scientific communities. Researchers studying human immunodeficiency virus/acquired immunodeficiency syndrome (HIV/AIDS), for example, have used retrospective (that is, backward-looking) studies of medical records in several ways. First, they were able to confirm that HIV/AIDS was, in fact, a new infectious disease. Second, by studying who had contracted the disease (for example, sexual behaviors, infants of infected mothers, and patients with hemophilia who had used contaminated blood products), they were able to determine how HIV is transmitted. Finally, they were able to track the spread of the disease within various population groups and geographic areas. At first all this research was done by studying the paper medical records of individual patients. However, the process of tracking the incidence and prevalence of this disease and others has become easier as more and more data have been digitized. Of course, in the United States and other developed countries, healthcare providers are required by law to report new cases of HIV/AIDS (and other communicable diseases) to the Centers for Disease Control and Prevention (CDC). The person's identity is held in strict confidence.

As you can see, the medical record has been used throughout history to benefit individual patients and to advance medical knowledge through research. Of course, there was the occasional country physician who never saw a need to keep records beyond those in his own head because he treated the same families in the same small communities generation after generation. However, failing to document a patient's care is no longer an option. Nowadays physicians are required to trade in their manila folders and outguides for scanners and mobile devices. In the following sections, we will explore documentation stored in the EHR and who is responsible for maintaining it.

Content of the Electronic Health Record

Each patient has his or her own health record or chart in the physician's office. This record tells the patient's health story. It is the source document for healthcare professionals and the documentation that provides evidence of care. Complete **documentation** in these records is vital to ensuring the highest level of care. The complexity of one's own health history is too overwhelming to memorize. Can you imagine trying to care for thousands of patients by memory? Impossible, and not an effective way to manage health. It's been said, "If it isn't documented, it never happened." Every patient encounter with the medical office must be tracked. Medical documentation of the events is the easiest and most effective way, and it's required by law. Therefore, maintaining and ensuring the accuracy of the medical record is one of the most important duties of the healthcare staff. The contents of the medical record may vary slightly from office to office, but most contain the types of documents outlined in the following text. Note, however, that there is some overlap among the categories—an insurance form, for example, is both an administrative and a legal document, and it may contain health information as well.

Clinical Information

The medical record is the primary source of information about the patient's medical history, such as immunization records, operative reports, and office visit notes. This information is gathered mostly during patient **encounters** (visits) with the physician. Over time, the stored clinical data are used to predict risk for disease, compare measurements and values against one another, and determine what is or is not effective for treatment of illness or other health problems. The more complete this record is, the better the care the provider can offer. Clinical information includes the following:

- Medication list (Figure 1-1)
- Allergies list
- Immunization records
- Laboratory reports
- Pathology reports
- Surgical reports
- Hospital records
- History and physical assessment findings
- Risk assessment
- Preventive services
- Progress notes
- Vital signs and growth charts
- Imaging test results, such as radiographs and magnetic resonance imaging (MRI) films

Figure 1-1
SCMO Medication list.

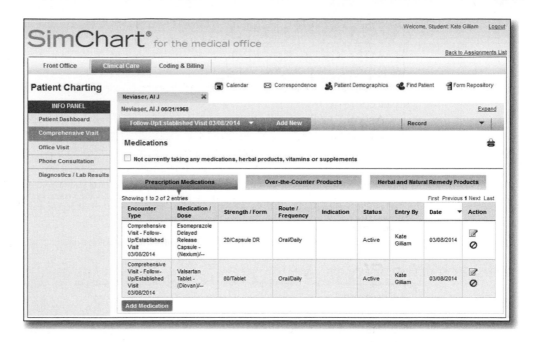

Administrative Information

In addition to clinical information, the administrative staff uses the medical record to perform front office activities such maintaining appointments, storing patient contact information, and creating patient correspondence. Administrative tasks also include the necessary coding and billing processes that keep the office doors open. Medical insurance policies are changing regularly, which makes gathering and storing current payer information important. Administrative information includes the following:

- Patient demographics
- Name of emergency contact person
- Patient correspondence
- Referral and consultation letters
- Prior authorizations
- Insurance information, copies of insurance cards
- Health Insurance Portability and Accountability Act (HIPAA) 5010 claims status
- Billing account ledgers
- Superbills
- Day sheets
- Appointment history
- Diagnosis and procedure codes

Legal Documents

On occasion a patient medical record may be used during court proceedings for malpractice suits. Thorough, accurate documentation helps prove what, when, and why something happened. For example, a complete record will show what information was provided to the patient and what decisions the patient or patient's family made concerning care options based on that information. Thus proper documentation is important to protect the practice as well as to ensure that the patient receives high-quality care.

Some legal forms that are part of the record, such as do not resuscitate (DNR) orders, may need to be accessed quickly for the medical team to know how to proceed in an emergency. The medical record, then, contains a variety of legal documents and, taken as a

Figure 1-2
SCMO General
Procedure form.

> # WALDEN-MARTIN
> FAMILY MEDICAL CLINIC
> 1234 ANYSTREET | ANYTOWN, ANYSTATE 12345
> PHONE 123-123-1234 | FAX 123-123-5678
>
> Student: Kate Gilliam
>
> ## General Procedure Consent
>
> **Patient Name:**   Thomas, Ken H   **Date:**   March 9, 2014
>
> The Doctor has discussed with you your condition and the recommended surgical or medical procedures to be performed. This discussion was intended to ensure that you had the opportunity to receive the information necessary to make a reasoned and informed decision whether or not to consent to the procedure. This document is written confirmation of the discussion and contain some of the more significant medical information discussed.
>
> **1. Based on this discussion, I understand the following condition may exist in my case:**
> Diverticulitis and colon polyps
>
> **2. I understand the procedure proposed for treating or diagnosing my condition is:**
> Colonscopy
>
> 3. I have been informed of the purpose and reasonable expected benefits of the proposed procedure, the possibility of success or failure, major problems of recuperation, the reasonably anticipated consequences if the procedure is not performed, and the available alternatives.
>
> 4. I understand that all surgical and therapeutic procedures involve some risks including pain, scarring, bleeding and infection.
>
> 5. I am aware that in the practice of medicine, other unexpected risks or complications not discussed may or may not further acknowledge that no guarantees or promises have been made to me concerning the results of any procedures. Although the benefits are judged to outweigh the risks, should any complications occur, any one of them could be permanent. I hereby voluntarily give my authority and consent to the doctor to perform the proposed procedure described above.
>
> 6. I have been given the opportunity to ask questions about my condition, alternative forms of treatment, risk treatment, the procedure to be used, and the risks and hazards involved. I believe I have sufficient information to give this informed consent.
>
> I understand I have read and fully understand the contents of this form, that the disclosure referred to above were made to me and that all blanks and statements requiring insertion or completion were filled in before I signed my name below.
>
> **Patient Signature:**   **Date:**
>
> **If a patient is a minor or unable to give consent,**
> **Signature of person authorized to consent for patient:**
>
> **Relationship to Patient:**

whole, can be considered a legal document in itself. Legal documentation includes the following:

- Medical records releases
- General procedure forms (Figure 1-2)
- HIPAA forms (notice of privacy practices)
- Advance directives
- Living wills
- Disclosure logs
- Healthcare power of attorney forms

WHO DOCUMENTS IN THE MEDICAL RECORD?

An individual who is responsible for inputting patient information into the medical record is called a *documenter.* This individual documents the patient's progress in chronologic order and records all new information or changes to the patient's health. The process of the documentation includes handwritten, dictated, structured data entry, or downloaded patient information.

In the past, some healthcare providers preferred to hand-write their notes. Caution had to be taken to ensure the notes were clear, complete, and easy to read. Handwritten

Figure 1-3
SCMO Patient
Information form.

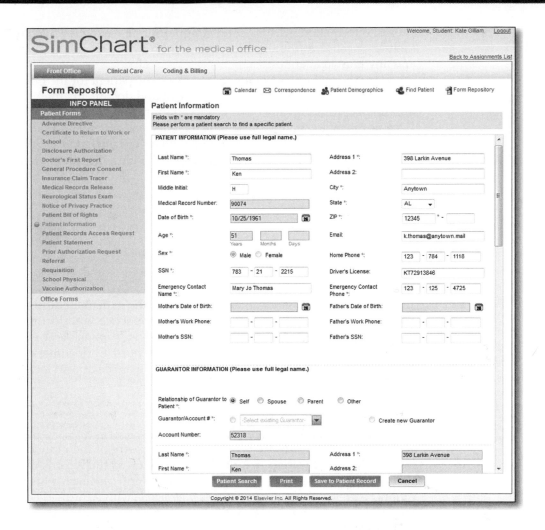

notes helped the provider avoid paying for transcription services, thereby reducing costs for the practice during the period of paper-based records. With the implementation of electronic systems, providers may choose to dictate a patient encounter directly into the medical record with the aid of voice recognition software. This is a computerized system that automatically converts voice into text as the physician speaks directly into a microphone. The error-free implementation of this software takes time because documenters must "train" the software to recognize the idiosyncrasies of their individual voices. Many medical software systems are moving from narrative-type notes to templates and **structured data entry.** These data are selected from a fixed field or database and make documentation from a mobile device easier to perform and provide standardization across all medical records in the system. Using these methods of documentation eliminates the need for a staff member to file physician documentation in the record or to transcribe taped information into the record.

Many different staff members within the physician's office contribute to the patient medical record. First, the receptionist or other member of the front-office staff records important basic data about the patient in preparation for consultation with and examination by the provider. This information is gathered using a **patient information form (PIF)** (Figure 1-3). The receptionist may be responsible for documenting notice of privacy practice (NPP) acknowledgments, the reason for patient visit, copayments, requests for prescription refills, and authorization to release medical records or obtain records from other physicians, as well as recording no-shows or cancellations of patient appointments.

The next documenter will generally be the medical assistant, who accompanies the patient to the examination room, records weight and vital signs, and notes preliminary clinical information, such as **chief complaint** (the reason for the patient's visit), history of the present illness (the duration and context of the chief complaint), medications taken, and any known allergies.

Once the medical assistant has prepared the patient for the physician's examination or consultation, the physician sees the patient and documents the history, examination findings, plan of care, and any other observations made during the patient encounter. The physician is the main documenter of the patient chart, and all additions to the patient medical record should be signed and approved with his or her signature. Many different healthcare providers may have documentation responsibilities, including the following:

- Primary care physician
- Physician's assistant
- Nurse practitioner
- Physical or occupational therapist
- Social worker
- Specialist
- Surgeon
- Medical biller

Each of these providers may contribute to the patient medical record in different ways. For example, the physical therapist's correspondence will document treatment plan and progress, whereas the primary care physician is responsible for coordinating all aspects of the patient's care. The medical biller may need to document the patient's insurance information and authorization numbers as well as file appeal letters and abstract data for claims submission.

WHO OWNS THE MEDICAL RECORD?

Patient medical records are considered the property of the individuals who created them. For example, a physician in a private practice owns the records created in his or her own practice. Records created at a hospital or a long-term care facility are the property of the institution. However, the patient owns the *information* within the medical record. In other words, the patient has a legal right to access or copy his or her own medical information at any time by signing a medical release form; however, the original copy of the record never leaves the facility that owns it. The patient also has the right to request restricted access, request amendments to errors, and obtain a list of disclosures (where information has traveled).

A medical practice may legally assign a fee for copying a medical record. This charge is based on the cost of preparation and production of the medical record. For example, in 2013, the MedChi (Maryland State Medical Society) specified that practices should assess a preparation fee of no more than $22.88, plus no more than 76 cents per page copied, plus the actual cost of shipping and handling. A physician's practice may withhold the copy if a patient has an unpaid balance on his or her account; however, patients cannot be charged pursuant to HIPAA standards. For example, if a patient believes false statements have been documented within his or her chart, the patient is able to obtain a copy of the medical records without having a fee applied. The physician's office may not withhold records from other physicians if doing so may be detrimental to the patient's care.

CRITICAL THINKING EXERCISE 1-1

Sherry Macken is a patient at the office where you work. She plans to move out of state and insists on taking her original (paper) patient medical chart with her. Although Ms. Macken has no unpaid balance on her account, the office manager refuses to release the record to her. Ms. Macken has just faxed a letter threatening to involve her brother-in-law, a personal injury lawyer whose ad appears on the back cover of the local phone book, if she does not receive her records within 1 week. Who legally owns the medical record, and how can this patient's situation be resolved amicably?

One exception to the patient's right to view his or her medical records is called the *doctrine of professional discretion.* This principle states that a physician can exercise his or her best judgment when deciding whether to share progress notes and clinical observations with a patient who is being treated for mental or emotional disturbances. The doctrine of professional discretion is intended to protect mentally or emotionally ill patients from any additional harm that viewing their medical records could cause. For example, fragile patients who are depressed or suicidal may be upset to read the practitioner's assessment of their unstable condition.

THE ELECTRONIC HEALTH RECORD

Traditionally, information pertaining to the patient's care in the medical office has been maintained using a paper-based chart. However, advancements in technology and government programs have caused a shift from paper-based records to digital ones. The **electronic health record (EHR),** simply put, is a patient medical record in an electronic format. Ideally, the EHR can exchange data freely with other computer systems, such as those of other healthcare providers, pharmacies, hospitals, laboratories, and insurance companies, creating one central EHR that is easily accessible to authorized parties yet secure from those who do not have the right to see it. That isn't always the case—but we'll talk more about that later in the chapter. For now, let's explore the features of a well-designed EHR.

The Eight Core Functions of an Electronic Health Records System

The Institute of Medicine (IOM) is a branch of the prestigious National Academy of Sciences, a not-for-profit organization. The IOM's mission is to offer objective, evidence-based advice on a broad range of healthcare topics to legislators, public health officials, healthcare providers, and representatives of the private sector who have a stake in the healthcare system. In 2003, the U.S. Department of Health and Human Services asked the IOM to create a set of standards for EHR systems. What, exactly, should an EHR accomplish? In response, the IOM outlined the following eight core functions of an EHR:

1. **Health information and data [management].** The EHR's cardinal function is to be a central repository for the patient's health information from a variety of sources.
2. **Results management.** Instituting an EHR system should make test results easily accessible.
3. **Order management.** The ability to order tests and prescribe medications electronically reduces errors and lowers costs.
4. **Decision support.** The EHR software should offer features that help clinicians manage patient care according to evidence-based treatment guidelines.
5. **Electronic communication and connectivity.** The chief advantage of an EHR system is that it allows all providers and institutions involved in a patient's care to communicate and share data efficiently, thereby improving the quality of the patient's care.
6. **Patient support.** Many EHR systems have tools for patient education, such as wound care instructions or guidelines for self-monitoring of blood glucose.
7. **Administrative processes.** Billing and scheduling can be handled electronically.
8. **Reporting and population health.** Diagnoses of infectious diseases can be reported confidentially to public health authorities, and researchers can access EHR databases to gather epidemiologic statistics (data on the incidence of a given disease and its prevalence within a certain population).

Transitioning from Paper to Electronic Records

The Bush administration first declared 2004–2014 "the decade of health information technology [HIT]" and established the Office of the National Coordinator for Health Information Technology (ONCHIT). Since then the Obama administration has continued to endorse and promote the universal use of EHR and **computerized provider order entry (CPOE)** in the Recovery Act of 2009 and the Affordable Care Act. These programs focus on improving coordination of care, reducing duplicative testing, and rewarding hospitals and providers for keeping patients healthier.

The transition of health information from paper-based records to electronic media has been slow but has had a dramatic increase recently. A nationwide survey conducted by DesRoche and colleagues showed that as of 2007–2008, only 17% of practices had adopted an EHR system. Data from the CDC's National Center for Health Statistics in 2012 reveal encouraging trends, with an implementation rate of 50% for physicians' offices and 80% for hospitals. Government programs offering financial incentives for EHR adoption have surely contributed to such trends (see Chapter 4).

EASING THE TRANSITION 1-1

Will e-Prescribing Solve the Problem of Medication Errors?

Physicians and bad handwriting go together like senators and lobbyists, cops and donuts, rock stars and rehab. But those uncrossed T's and scrawled numbers are more than just a cliché. Illegible handwriting is downright dangerous. An estimated 1.5 million medication errors occur each year, thousands of which can be attributed to sloppy script. Hespan can be mistaken for Heparin, or Norcuron can look like Narcan. In fact, the manufacturer of the Alzheimer's drug Reminyl changed the drug's name because two people died after being given the diabetes drug Amaryl.

The problem goes beyond drug names, though. Hurriedly written 2's can look like 7's, or 0's can resemble 6's, leading to dosage errors. Abbreviations are another source of peril. For example, the abbreviation "qhs" on a prescription, which means "taken at the hour of sleep [bedtime]," can look like "qhr," which means "taken every hour." Seven thousand deaths each year are attributable to these kinds of medication errors.

A number of solutions have been proposed for the problem. The Institute for Safe Medication Practices (ISMP) publishes a continually updated list of sound-alike medications and a list of dangerous abbreviations, symbols, and dose designations, along with suggested alternatives. The ISMP recommends, for example, that "nightly" be substituted for "qhs." In addition, safety advocates urge prescribers to write a brief description of the diagnosis, such as "for Alzheimer's," directly on the prescription as an additional cross-check for the pharmacist to confirm that he or she is dispensing the right medication. Patients, too, should take an active role in preventing errors by checking prescription labels, reading the leaflets or product inserts accompanying their prescriptions, and consulting with the pharmacist if the pills they're given are a different size, shape, or color from those previously dispensed for the same prescription.

But is e-prescribing (CPOE) the real solution to poor penmanship? The answer is a qualified yes. After all, typewritten drug names and dosages are always legible. The VA, which has converted entirely to EHR systems, issues more than 230 million prescriptions a year and claims an accuracy rate of nearly 100%. The VA checks hospital patients' prescriptions against a bar code on their wristbands to make sure the drug being dispensed will not react adversely with the patients' other medications. By using built-in clinical decision support tools, the EHR system makes sure the drug is compatible with the patient's diagnosis. The system also produces automatic warnings if the dosage entered is beyond the range normally prescribed.

According to an annual survey on EHR systems conducted by the American Academy of Family Physicians, physicians are enthusiastic about e-prescribing, ranking it as one of the top five advantages of EHR systems. However, the e-prescribing function isn't foolproof. A study published in the *Journal of the American Medical Association (JAMA)* found that the use of EHR systems actually facilitated 22 new kinds of prescribing errors unrelated to legibility. For instance, the prescriber can still click on the wrong medication when selecting from an alphabetical list, or choose, say, a tablet instead of the liquid formulation of a drug. Another kind of error occurred, the researchers found, when prescribers viewed a pharmacy inventory on the screen (indicating, for instance, that the 200-mg tablets of a given medication were in stock) and mistook it for prescribing guidelines that help physicians determine the customary dosage of a drug. Because it may take as many as 20 screens to view a single patient's medications, errors also occurred in failing to

Continued

EASING THE TRANSITION 1-2—cont'd

discontinue a previously prescribed drug when a replacement drug is ordered. A medication can even be prescribed to the wrong patient when one prescriber fails to log off the system at a shared computer terminal.

Nevertheless, the advantage of an electronic system over paper in reducing medication errors is undeniable. Even the aforementioned *JAMA* study concluded that EHR systems are less subject to error caused by sound-alike drug names and mistaken dosages. The report also concluded that the CPOE systems built in to EHR systems are able to reduce under- and overprescribing and can easily be linked to drug interaction warnings and clinical decision support systems that help ensure accuracy. Although we should be aware that e-prescribing is not a cure-all and has generated unexpected kinds of errors, we must acknowledge that it nevertheless represents a dramatic advance toward the goal of keeping patients safe.

As healthcare becomes more and more complex, physicians have tried to find ways to make patient information more accessible and organized. The EHR aims to accomplish this. HIPAA stipulates nationwide adoption of EHR systems by 2014 (the details of HIPAA and meaningful use programs are discussed throughout this text). Building the necessary infrastructure has taken years and required a capital investment of more than $150 billion, plus nearly $50 billion per year in operating expenses.

What Is the Difference Between an Electronic Health Record and an Electronic Medical Record?

As the concept of the EHR evolved over time, a distinction was sometimes made between the terms *EHR* and *electronic medical record (EMR)*. The EMR was said to be an electronic patient record created and maintained by a medical practice or hospital, whereas the EHR was said to be an interconnected aggregate of all the patient's health records, culled from multiple providers and healthcare facilities. In other words, the EMR was said to be a component of the EHR. In practice, however, the line between these terms has blurred to the point that they are now used virtually interchangeably, although there has been a shift toward EHR as the preferred term. This makes sense. After all, the purpose of converting records from paper to an electronic format is ultimately to create a single record for each patient that allows providers and facilities to update, access, and share information efficiently. Using the term *EHR* reflects the healthcare industry's optimism that this goal will be met in the foreseeable future, whereas continuing to make a distinction between the terms perpetuates the idea that each medical practice maintains its own records. In this text, we will refer to electronic patient records, whether created by a medical practice or by a hospital or other facility, as EHR systems.

Electronic Health Records Software

A variety of EHR software systems are on the market. They should all be able to perform the eight core functions as discussed previously. In addition, they should be certified by the **Certification Commission for Healthcare Information Technology (CCHIT).** The CCHIT issues standards for what each software system should be able to accomplish. Although the systems still may not be compatible, this standardization of functionality is a necessary first step toward becoming interconnected.

Most EHR systems have the same basic functionality, with differences in task execution, navigation, work flow, and so forth. Because their fundamental features are similar, the user can adapt to different systems with little difficulty. The SimChart for the Medical Office (SCMO) is a web-based EHR that has real functionality used in physicians' offices and outpatient facilities while giving students a safe, academic learning environment. Its features are demonstrated throughout this text.

Basic Functions

Commercial EHR systems have the following fundamental capabilities:

- Progress notes function
- Documentation using free text, predefined clinical templates, user-defined clinical templates, or clinical macros
- Provider review of incoming lab data, reports
- Patient correspondence
- Storage of office forms (incident reports, inventory, petty cash)
- Images and report attachment function
- Electronic signature insertion
- Prescription (CPOE) templates that provide dosage, suggest alternatives, list prices, and cross-check prescriptions for drug interactions, patient allergies, and availability in the formulary
- Fax and messaging functions to transmit prescriptions directly from the EHR to the patient's pharmacy
- Reminders that the patient is due for a screening or other health maintenance test or procedure
- Vital signs data capture
- Patient portal
- Importation of lab data from an outside or in-house lab, using industry-standard formats
- Automatic flagging of abnormal data and test results
- Intraoffice messaging and email functions
- Summary and print functions

Clinical Decision Support

An advanced feature called **clinical decision support (CDS)** allows practitioners to tailor the care of an individual patient by making sure it adheres to published guidelines for the patient's specific diagnoses. Clinical decision support tools allow providers to do the following:

- Ensure that the patient's care complies with established screening recommendations for the diseases for which he or she is at risk (colon cancer or glaucoma, for instance). EHR systems analyze patient data, such as age and gender, in order to produce automated reminders for mammograms, Pap smears, colonoscopies, diabetic retinopathy exams, and other screening tests and procedures.
- Plan treatment in accordance with evidence-based treatment guidelines (for heart failure or hepatitis, for example). The practitioner can make more accurate and timely diagnoses with the aid of advice automatically generated by the EHR system based on the patient's clinical data.
- Generate patient data reports and summaries.
- Complete documentation templates specific to the patient's diagnosis, such as knee pain or kidney disease.
- Perform database searches to identify patients who meet specific criteria, such as those within a particular age range who have a given diagnosis, in order to ensure that they are receiving the recommended care and screening. For example, it is recommended that pregnant women with diabetes be closely monitored for diabetic retinopathy for 1 year postpartum because pregnancy can accelerate the development of this ophthalmologic complication. The clinician could query the EHR database to produce a list of women in the practice with diabetes who have given birth within the last year and who have not received a diabetic retinopathy screening in 3 months or longer. These patients could then be contacted and immediately referred to a retina specialist.

The CDS tools work, however, only if providers take advantage of them. A statewide study of Massachusetts physicians found that fewer than half of them whose EHR systems offered CDS actually used it. Furthermore, if information is not entered properly, some CDS functions are less effective. For example, one practice decided to use its EHR system to identify all female patients ages 50 to 65 who had not had a mammogram in a year or longer. Because of data that had been entered in an improper format, 15% of patients who met those criteria were not found during the initial search.

In addition, clinicians may ignore system-generated advice either because they're busy or because they prefer to rely on their own judgment and experience. Some practices may not even install this function, especially if there is no financial incentive for delivering care in conformity with established protocols, such as evidence-based guidelines for prescribing antibiotics prophylactically (in other words, to prevent an infection) before a patient undergoes a gastrointestinal endoscopy procedure.

Proponents of the advanced tools say that CDS allows them to focus more on patient communication skills and their ability to make critical decisions. Instead of spending all of their time trying to memorize treatment protocols, physicians are able to focus on the patient examination and the needs of the individual. On December 11, 2013, legislators introduced the Excellence in Diagnostic Imaging Utilization Act of 2013, which requires the use of clinical guidance tools (CDS tools) when ordering diagnostic testing. Along with this act, any provider who wishes to receive Meaningful Use Incentive Program dollars is required to implement at least one CDS element (or rule) for patients. Under the requirement, the clinical decision support can help providers:

- Share best practices regarding the treatment and diagnosis of disease
- Reduce the amount of testing ordered by physicians and then denied by insurance companies
- Improve clinical outcomes and reduce the number of misdiagnoses
- Reduce costs from unnecessary testing
- Improve patient safety

CRITICAL THINKING EXERCISE 1-2

During Dr. Martin's visit with Mr. Hickman, he discovers that the patient has gained 22 pounds since his visit 4 months ago and that his triglycerides are high. Dr. Martin wants to check the recommended adult dosage of the cholesterol-lowering drug he intends to prescribe; calculate the patient's body mass index (BMI) based on his sex, height, and weight; and give Mr. Hickman a patient education brochure explaining the link between physical inactivity, being overweight, and type 2 diabetes. Which of these functions can he accomplish using his practice's EHR system? How would Dr. Martin go about gathering this information? How might the use of CDS tools help manage Mr. Hickman's diagnosis?

Practice Management Software

The EHR lies at the heart of the modern digital medical office, but most medical practices choose to kick it up a notch by using a fully integrated EHR and practice management system, such as that offered in the SCMO. **Practice management software (PMS)** allows electronic management of the business side of the practice. It allows efficient handling of all front-office administrative procedures, including entering patient demographics, tracking billing and insurance information, scheduling appointments, and processing payments for patient visits. Let's take a look at what integrated practice management software has to offer.

Patient Demographics

Practice management software compiles all of a patient's demographic information—socioeconomic data such as age, sex, marital status, education, occupation, and perhaps even religious preference—within the EHR. When patients present to the physician's

Figure 1-4
SCMO Patient
Demographics screen.

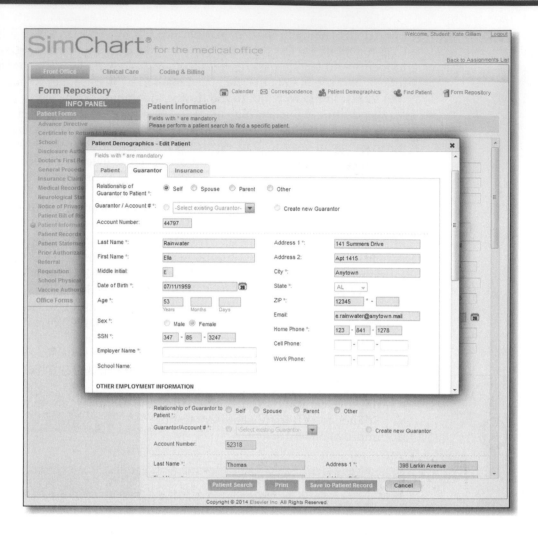

office, they are asked to fill out a **patient information form (PIF)** that asks them to provide their identifying and contact information, including name, home and work addresses, phone numbers, email address, and Social Security number. Some questions about clinical issues, such as reason for visit (chief complaint), and administrative matters, such as insurance information, are included on the form as well. The Patient Demographics tool in the SCMO stores all of the information on three tabs: Patient, Guarantor, and Insurance (Figure 1-4).

Billing and Insurance Information

A scanned copy of the patient's medical insurance card(s), if he or she is insured, should be obtained at each visit. Information should be obtained about the patient's type of medical insurance (for example, workers' compensation or Medicare), insurance carrier, claims submission address and phone number, policy and group numbers, and required copayment. A **copayment** is the amount of money a patient is contracted to pay out of pocket at each visit. Figure 1-5 shows a sample insurance card.

Appointment Scheduling

Patients who need to see a healthcare provider are usually asked to make an appointment—a specific time and date reserved to meet with the healthcare professional (physician, physician's assistant, or nurse practitioner). The healthcare professional will examine the patient and consult with him or her about the chief complaint (which, as noted above, is the patient's main reason for seeking healthcare services). Depending on

Figure 1-5
Sample insurance cards.

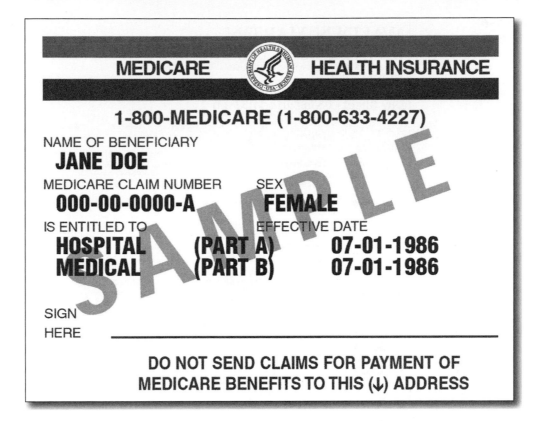

office policy, the provider may schedule patients in a variety of ways. The most common method of appointment scheduling is a fixed schedule, according to which the patient is asked to appear in the office at a specific date and time. Typical fixed appointments range from 10 to 30 minutes for acutely ill established patients to 1 hour for new-patient visits. An established patient is one who has been seen by a member of the healthcare team within the past 3 years. A new patient is one who has not been seen in the past 3 years by any member of the office. Electronic appointments integrated into the EHR allow quick search of available appointments, easy rescheduling, documentation of cancellations, and quick links to the patient's clinical record. (We talk more about these functions in Chapter 5.)

Figure 1-6
SCMO Day Sheet.

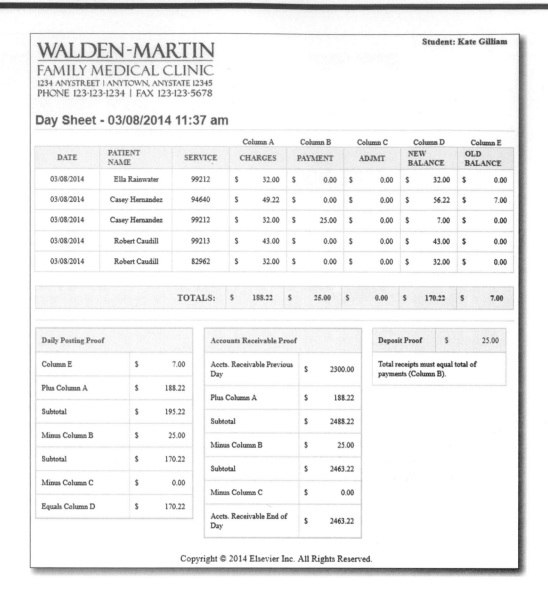

Advanced Accounting Procedures

Patient accounting is important to the success of the healthcare practice. Accounting procedures performed by practice management software include management and creation of patient statements, generation of day sheets, and completion of HIPAA 5010 claim format. An **account ledger** is a document that contains a responsible payer's name (guarantor), patient's identifying and contact information, appointment details, payments made, insurance reimbursements received, balance owed, and amount outstanding. The billing account ledger is a list of the outstanding balances for all appointments up to the current date. A **day sheet,** or day journal, is a register of daily business transactions (Figure 1-6). The day sheet is a system of checks and balances for the office as it prepares to make deposits into the bank. The account ledger and day sheet are both ways of documenting patients' financial information.

After the patient's financial information has been documented for the medical office, a claim must be submitted to a third-party payer. A **third-party payer** is someone other than the patient, spouse, parent, or guardian who is responsible for paying all or part of the patient's medical expenses. In most cases, the third party is a medical insurance company. A HIPAA 5010 is a standard electronic format that speeds claims processing for physicians and suppliers (Figure 1-7).

Most certified EHR systems can perform these functions. The billing functionality of the EHR is discussed in greater detail in Chapter 7.

Figure 1-7
SCMO HIPAA 5010

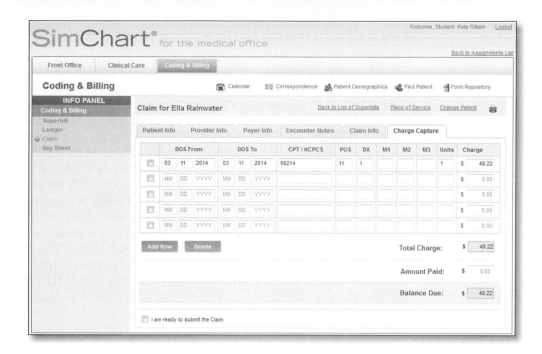

ADVANTAGES OF ELECTRONIC HEALTH RECORDS

Improved Quality and Continuity of Care

It is estimated that patients who visit a physician for a specific condition have about a 50/50 chance of getting the recommended evidence-based care. With complete and immediate access to patient records, however, practitioners can provide better and faster treatment, raising the level of both medical care and personal attention from the healthcare team. Multiple physicians and healthcare workers are able to access and view the EHR at one time.

One of the most important ways in which an EHR can improve quality is by ensuring **continuity of care.** Contemporary healthcare—and the fast pace of modern life in general—requires complex patient histories to be accommodated quickly and accurately. Providers must be able to plan and coordinate care efficiently in order to ensure high quality and avoid duplication of services. To do so they must be able to communicate with each other on the double, without waiting for phone calls to be returned or copies to be made and faxed. Ideally, patients should be able to move from one physician to another—for a second opinion, for example—without having to visit or call physicians, hospitals, imaging centers, and labs to collect their records on paper or film.

Let's look at a few situations in which this kind of continuity is especially important.

Managing Patients with Chronic Conditions

First, continuity of care is critical when multiple specialists must plan and coordinate the treatment of a patient with a serious chronic condition like Parkinson's disease, hepatitis C, or prostate cancer. Specialists must be able to communicate lab findings, medications prescribed, operative notes, and other information within a hospital, assisted living center, hospice, or other healthcare setting. In addition, the patient's primary care provider must be able to track, organize, store, and retrieve the information so that the patient will receive competent follow-up when treatment ends. The physician will want to know, for instance, how many treatment cycles are planned, which tests have been performed, whether the patient has any new mobility restrictions, what medications have been prescribed, and whether the patient has experienced confusion, memory loss, sexual dysfunction, or other side effects.

Disaster Preparedness and Response

Continuity of care is also crucial in effective disaster preparedness and response. The advantage for an emergency department or field triage unit of gaining immediate access to a person's medical record is obvious. The more victims whose records can be accessed at or near the time and place of a disaster, the better. But the benefit of EHR systems extends beyond this immediate need. Electronic records are generally backed up by a secure web-based system and thus can be retrieved even when the computers at a medical practice or hospital are destroyed by fire, flood, or other means. In fact, more and more EHR systems are being offered completely over the Internet to their subscribers. In this respect, EHR systems are actually more durable than paper records. Victims of Hurricane Katrina who received their medical care from the Veterans Health Administration (VA), for instance, received better, more timely care than those whose records were destroyed in the hurricane and its aftermath. The benefits of EHR systems continue to be seen in subsequent events as well. As part of the Hurricane Sandy preparation, hospitals were able to plan for patient care by contacting patients and having generators in place to operate their systems. Reflection of these events has revealed three health IT must-haves during natural disasters: on-site safety, off-site data, and accessibility. All of these are possible with EHR systems.

Increased Efficiency

An EHR system makes patient information readily available to healthcare practitioners and support staff. Providers who use the EHR include physicians, nurses, medical assistants, administrative assistants, medical records management personnel, medical coders, and medical billing specialists. Using the EHR saves time. Instead of hunting down a misfiled chart in a large file room or conducting an archeologic dig through the pile on Dr. Martin's desk, the EHR puts the patient record right at your fingertips. Time that was wasted in the past is now freed to perform other duties in the office. In addition, much less office space is required to store the records, providing extra space for examination rooms, offices, medical equipment, and other uses.

Improved Documentation

Documentation provides legal evidence of competent patient care and serves as an invaluable research tool. **Electronic transcription** using structured data entry (drop-down menus and automatic sentence builders) eliminates the need for handwritten notes, which tend to be riddled with errors. These structured data entry tools allow the physician or other documenter to select from preconstructed options (templates) or choices within a record or document. By stringing these choices together, progress notes, letters, medication lists, and other documentation can be accomplished electronically. Forcing the documenter to use selected choices within the screen's template eliminates the need to free-key the work and can be easier when working with mobile devices.

This form of data entry essentially eliminates illegible handwriting and incomplete notes. Illegible handwriting can lead to errors in reporting, diagnosis, treatment, and billing procedures. However, in earlier EMR systems, using this tool was sometimes more time consuming than documenting on paper. One physician found that it took more than a minute and a half and 17 clicks on yes/no and drop-down menu choices to document one patient's back pain diagnosis. Yet it took just 41 seconds to handwrite his documentation for the same diagnosis into the patient's paper chart. Certified EHR systems have recognized this inconvenience and worked to make documentation more user friendly.

The EHR also can link records electronically. This is useful in patient education, allowing healthcare providers to compare test results or graph a comparison of patient weight and blood pressure.

Electronic documentation reduces data entry errors and helps ensure a complete patient record. Documentation that is clear, complete, accurate, and legible is extremely important to the success of the EHR and to the medical practice.

Why Document Properly?

1. To avoid delay of reimbursement or denial of claims because medical necessity of services provided has not been proved.
2. To comply with insurance companies' and accreditation companies' enforcement of documentation guidelines for healthcare facilities.
3. To aid the work of investigators and regulators when legal issues arise, including subpoenas of medical records in court cases and state investigations.
4. To protect the practice in case a malpractice suit is brought.
5. To facilitate communication among healthcare providers.
6. To establish evidence of care.

Easier Accessibility at the Point of Care

The EHR is intended to make patient information more accessible to healthcare providers. The availability of the EHR is limited only by privacy and security measures. As we know, patients don't get sick only during regular office hours. An injured or acutely ill patient may present to the emergency department at 3 AM. The availability of an interconnected EHR allows the medical team to access the patient's health history immediately. Having the entire health record at their fingertips gives medical personnel a broad, accurate picture of the patient's health status and decreases delays in initiating care.

Better Security

Passwords increase security and allow only authorized individuals to access patient medical records. Many healthcare facilities require their users to change their passwords periodically. Tracking or **auditing** user access reveals a history, like a trail of breadcrumbs, of who has accessed the record, what users have viewed, and who modified any given patient record. Auditing is usually performed by a member of office management and can be done to determine whether an employee has accessed information inappropriately. Violating a patient's privacy is illegal under HIPAA and is grounds for immediate termination of employment.

Reduced Expenses

As discussed earlier, an EHR system eliminates the need for most transcription, which can cost an office thousands of dollars each year. Records are stored electronically, dramatically reducing the need for paper storage facilities. Using an EHR system also reduces duplication of services, such as tests that have already been performed at another facility. Using CDS functionality, EHR systems can also flag any tests ordered that might be unnecessary given the patient's diagnosis and clinical data.

Improved Job Satisfaction

Transitioning to an EHR system, at best, tries everyone's patience and, at worst, brings the office to a near standstill as providers and staff key patient data into electronic files and learn to use the new interface. However, once an EHR system has been adopted and fully implemented within an office, most say they would never go back to paper. A 2012 EHR user satisfaction survey conducted by the American Academy of Family Physicians reported that 75% of physician users were happy with their EHR system (total sample size of 3088).

Providers

Those directly involved in patient care, such as physicians and nurse practitioners, feel more confident that they are delivering high-quality care after an EHR system is implemented.

For example, if a drug is recalled from the market, every patient in the practice to whom that drug has been prescribed can be identified by executing a simple computer search that takes just seconds. The patients can then be quickly notified, and either a prescription for a substitute drug can be called in to the patient's pharmacy (whose phone number is listed in the EHR) or an appointment can be scheduled. In fact, the VA used clinical data, such as laboratory values, stored in patients' EHR systems to identify chronic kidney disease in one third of those with diabetes even though they had no symptoms. Small practices can conduct this kind of analysis on a smaller scale. They can also deliver better quality at the point of care.

A survey of Massachusetts physicians showed that those whose practices had adopted EHR systems were less likely to feel demoralized about the state of the medical profession, reported significantly more positive views about how computers might affect healthcare quality, and were far more likely to believe that computers have a positive effect on communication with their patients.

Staff

Support staff, too, feel better able to manage a busy practice when an EHR system is in place. The software provides neat, standardized forms on which to record phone messages and transmit them to physicians. A logical, built-in workflow allows prescription refills to be handled safely and efficiently. Laboratory reports, results of imaging studies, and similar data are handled in a consistent fashion. Letters to patients can be expedited using customizable templates. Staff members say they spend less time chasing charts, clarifying prescription orders for pharmacies, and performing billing, coding, and transcription tasks. Communication with providers requires fewer interruptions during patient appointments, which makes everyone happier—including the patients.

Improved Patient Satisfaction

Patients appreciate the increased efficiency an EHR system offers. A 2013 survey by the Employee Benefits Research Institute revealed that 82% of Americans say they believe they receive better quality of care from a physician who uses EHRs. When the medical office uses an EHR system, patients tend to have greater confidence that their messages will be returned quickly and that their call-in prescriptions will be refilled promptly. Patients appreciate having access to their health information via a patient portal, ease of appointment scheduling, and receiving test results. Office visits are more productive because the physician can access the data he or she needs just by tapping on the screen of a tablet PC. The physician no longer has to retrieve a file or book to look up dosages or thumb through the patient's chart looking for stray information.

A study by Johnson and colleagues concluded that computerized documentation had a positive effect on interaction between physicians and parents during pediatric visits. In particular, physicians using EHR systems posed more open-ended questions and had a conversational style that was more patient centered than that of physicians who were not using electronic documentation. A study by Ventres and colleagues found that patients as well as physicians liked EHR systems that can be displayed on a flat-screen computer monitor with a mobile arm, so that providers can discuss the information in the patients' own charts. Most physicians preferred to alternate between entering data and interviewing the patient, creating a collaborative physician-patient-computer interaction. The authors of the study observed that the EHR becomes a reliable "third party" in the physician-patient conversation.

DISADVANTAGES OF ELECTRONIC HEALTH RECORDS

Of course, any technologic advance comes with a downside, and EHR systems are no exception. Let's take a look at some of the kinks that still need to be worked out, as well as some disadvantages of EHR systems that are likely to remain permanently.

Lack of Interoperability

Compatibility standards have not yet been universally applied to ensure that systems can interact with, or "talk to," one another. This capability is known as **interoperability.** The concept is similar to the interoperability of some computer operating systems and is one of the core functions of certified electronic health record technology. Certified EHR systems are compatible with specific laboratory, pharmacy, and hospital networks. However, not all EHR systems are compatible with one another. When information is received in an incompatible format, it must be hand-keyed into the record, or the appropriate template must be filled out. One small practice found that it took 13 mouse clicks just to enter mammography data for one patient.

This lack of uniformity has become a real dilemma both for individual patients and for the U.S. healthcare system as a whole. If a hospital uses a different EHR system from that of a patient's primary care physician, the patient's health records may not be available to the hospital, or vice versa. Let's say a patient experiences a bowel perforation. Emergency personnel at the trauma center request a list of medications from the patient's physician. The list has to be faxed to the trauma center and then keyed in to the patient's record there because the physician's EHR system can't communicate with the hospital's EHR interface. As the patient is treated, his or her operative summary, progress notes, radiographs, and psychiatric consultation reports must be snail-mailed to his or her primary care physician.

As you can see, EHR systems reduce paperwork within an office, but until they become interoperable, communication among various treating healthcare providers, pharmacies, and allied healthcare workers will be limited. The healthcare system must solve the problem of interoperability because it increases costs, decreases efficiency, introduces opportunities for error (when information is re-keyed), and discourages small providers from adopting EHR systems.

Cost

One of the chief barriers to adopting an EHR system is the steep start-up cost in terms of both time and money. Nearly 70% of all interactions between physicians and patients occur in practices that have four physicians or fewer. These practices are small businesses that, just like any other, must control costs, weigh the benefits of capital investment (such as an EHR system), and decide how staff time will be spent.

Financial Investment

The medical office must buy the software system or subscribe to an EHR vendor (see Chapter 4) to record and store patient charts. The cost of EHR implementation depends on the type of system being used. Recent estimates of "in-house" software are around $37,000 to start up. Web-based EHRs (software as a service [SAAS]) are estimated at $34,000 for the first year. Customizing the EHR for a particular medical office is very costly. In addition, hardware upgrades may be necessary to accommodate the new software.

The cost of these investments is borne by the practice, yet insurance companies and other third parties may benefit most from the upgrades. Grants and incentives may be available to offset the cost. For example, one large health system in Washington State offers $2 per visit, as well as other incentives, for each patient's record that is handled electronically. Disincentives to remain with paper charting have entered the mix, too. By federal law, a reimbursement penalty is in place for physicians who do not use an electronic prescribing system for their Medicare patients.

Many providers are concerned that they could purchase one system, only to have it become obsolete if another platform becomes the standard. It is important for providers to purchase only EHR systems certified by CCHIT. Many practices have been waiting for the bugs to be worked out and for interconnectivity to improve. However, publication of the CCHIT standards seems to have been a tipping point, after which the conversion to EHR systems began to gather momentum. Those who had been wavering apparently have begun to feel more secure about making the investment and are being required to do so to maintain current reimbursement levels.

Time

Additional costs include the expense of lost productivity while staff members are training instead of doing their normal jobs and the cost of paying for the training sessions, although the latter are often provided free by the software company as a purchasing incentive. Finally, converting all charts to the electronic format is costly and time consuming because it takes staff away from their normal jobs and limits the number of patients who can be seen during the transition. All information in a patient's paper chart must be entered into the EHR before the electronic system can be used for that patient. Depending on whether a phased implementation is used, this process can divert resources from patient care and office support functions for weeks or even months.

Employee Resistance

Employees who have been part of the medical office for an extended time may resist the conversion to an EHR. They may be concerned that the EHR is difficult to use and may not be familiar with computer technology. Physicians may feel as if they are doing "busywork" that they used to be able to delegate to staff. Those who plan to retire within 5 or 10 years will endure all the pain of the transition but have many fewer years during which to gain from the system's implementation.

The EHR changes the way the administrative and clinic processes are done in the office. Job responsibilities and duties often need to be modified. For example, the role of the file clerk changes dramatically. No longer will this staff member have to pull charts or file documents. Everything is done digitally. Perhaps this person will take on new duties, such as importing documents from other providers and facilities or focusing on maintenance of the EHR system.

The medical staff, including physicians, will have to take additional steps and time to ensure that proper documentation is done. This can distract EHR users from patient care as they try to learn the new technology.

EASING THE TRANSITION 1-2

Generation Gap: Training the Office "Dinosaur"

Your practice has finally decided to adopt an EHR system, and everyone in your practice is pumped with excitement about making the switch—well, nearly everyone. One of the senior physicians, Dr. Crabtree, refuses to take part, insisting that he'll continue to maintain paper records for his patients.

This scenario is familiar in just about every office that has exchanged paper charting for the great unknown of electronic records. In fact, businesses of all kinds are faced with the problem of workers who are uncomfortable using new technology. Some of these late adopters seem to take a certain pride in remaining "dinosaurs." But does adopting an EHR system have to lead to generational skirmishes, with seniors on one side and everyone else on the other?

The term "computer literacy"—which is really too vague to be useful—has given way to the idea of "networked workers." A networked or wired worker is likely to take advantage of electronic devices, such as cell phones, laptop computers, and tablet PCs, both at home and at work. According to data from the Pew Internet and American Life project, 86% of American workers use the Internet or email at least occasionally. Nearly half of all employed Americans have worked from home using a computer. But only about half of working adults ages 60 to 69 go online. (This proportion is growing, but only because aging Baby Boomers, who tend to be avid networked workers, are entering the 60+ age group.)

Continued

EASING THE TRANSITION 1-2—cont'd

Older healthcare personnel—physicians, nurses, and office workers alike—may perceive computerized health records systems as complex, inflexible, or even unnecessary. They may have heard horror stories from their adult children and others about having their hard drives wiped out or becoming the victims of phishing scams. Researchers at Fidelity Investments have coined the term "cautious clickers" to describe the computer behavior of older generations. They move from screen to screen with extreme hesitation, fearing that one false click will crash the system or that they won't remember how to get back to where they were. They linger over instructions and become frustrated trying to scroll and navigate windows and screens.

So how can the networked workers bring the late adopters on board? Here are a few tips on winning over the Dr. Crabtree in your office:

1. Avoid teasing your reluctant convert. The person may already feel left out or be embarrassed by a lack of computer skills, and rubbing it in won't help. Offer a separate training session for employees with varied levels of computer comfort.

2. Remind Dr. Crabtree how much he relies on older technologies that were once considered cutting edge—calculators, cell phones, and medical imaging devices such as MRI machines, for instance.

3. Appeal to Dr. Crabtree's sense of fairness and teamwork. If he refuses to use the technology, others will have to take up the slack. And besides, using the EHR system makes it easier for other physicians to cover for him when he is out of the office.

4. Offer to provide additional training as he learns to use the system. If possible, have someone who knows the software shadow him for a couple of days—or longer—to mentor him as he gets his feet wet. Reassure him that he can come on in—the water's fine!

5. Explain how an EHR system can enhance the quality of patient care with CDS tools by sending automatic cancer screening reminders, matching cardiac patients with American Heart Association treatment protocols, and so on. With patients' permission, let Dr. Crabtree observe another physician to see how EHR systems can be displayed on-screen and used as a partner, of sorts, during consultations.

6. Keep your language simple, and avoid using acronyms, abbreviations, and computer terminology that might confuse him. For example, don't assume Dr. Crabtree knows what it means to IM, to download an image, or to execute a search. Remember that he probably won't understand what things like drop-down menus and dialog boxes are.

7. Figure out what motivates your unwired colleague and appeal to his self-interest. For example, if Dr. Crabtree often stays late at the office, show him how the EHR system will allow him to work from home. If he has 11 grandchildren, remind him how easy it will be to stay in touch with them once he learns to use email and share files. Computer skills are transferable, after all!

8. Above all, be patient! The Fidelity researchers found that it takes people older than age 55 nearly 50% longer than their younger counterparts to complete a given computer task. It's likely that any of us would have the same hesitation and apprehension if we'd been born a few decades earlier. A little genuine understanding goes a long way.

Regimentation

The standardization built in to almost any computer program cannot accommodate idiosyncrasies. Practitioners who formerly had different ways of handling their charting must suddenly adapt to a regimented system that pigeonholes tasks. Despite evidence indicating potential improvements in quality of care, some physicians complain that EHR systems rely too heavily on check boxes and quantitative data rather than on descriptive terms and narrative. They believe that the need to standardize documentation takes the art out of the science of medicine.

One older internist, referring to the electronically prepared reports he receives from other physicians, lamented the lack of any evidence of the provider's reasoning or the patient's emotions, saying that the templates produce "a skeleton of data without the meat." This concern was echoed by participants in a study by Ventres and colleagues. They worried that EHR notes lack narrative depth, creating "cookie cutter" charts and forcing them to practice "cookbook medicine." However, other providers who took part in the study noted that the built-in clinical protocols gave them a quick and effective way to apply evidence-based algorithms to individual patients. Perhaps as systems evolve and as providers adapt to using them, EHR interfaces will offer more opportunities to enter descriptive data and providers will be more willing to take advantage of these features.

CRITICAL THINKING EXERCISE 1-3

Dr. Gregorio is in practice with his daughter, a new physician, who is urging him to make the switch from paper to electronic records. The elder Dr. Gregorio believes his modest practice is too small to require such a system. Besides, he argues, his patients find it reassuring to see him take notes on paper. The younger Dr. Gregorio thinks it's her father, not his patients, who are reluctant to change. How could you encourage the two Dr. Gregorios to purchase an EHR system? What do you think would be the pros and cons of purchasing the system for a small practice?

Security Gaps

With the implementation of HIPAA, interest in protecting patient security and privacy has been heightened. A patient's medical records must remain confidential. However, it may be possible for individuals to penetrate EHR systems despite security precautions and then sell, release, or change confidential information. This has some patients worried about how safe and confidential their electronic medical records really are. Security standards are outlined by HIPAA and the Health Information Technology for Economic and Clinical Health (HITECH) Act; both work to streamline methods of implementation. Power outages, viruses, backup procedures, and computer freezes and crashes pose other safety and security concerns for medical offices using EHR systems. System security is one important step to proving compliance with the Meaningful Use program, and providers must prove that standard and compliance programs are in place (see Chapter 3).

✔ SECURITY CHECKPOINT 1-1

Celebrity Health Records Become Tabloid Fodder: Should You Care?

Checkout-line tabloids are willing to pay big bucks to snoop into celebrities' personal lives, and their health records have become more vulnerable now that they can often be accessed electronically on the networks of healthcare institutions that employ thousands of people. The health records of Britney Spears, Farrah Fawcett, Maria Shriver, Tom Cruise, Brad Pitt, and Paula Abdul have allegedly been subject to recent privacy invasions. Spears's records, for instance, may have been viewed without her consent when she gave birth to her first child and when she was hospitalized for a psychiatric evaluation. In 2013, six Cedar-Sinai Medical Center employees were fired for inappropriately accessing the patient record of Kim Kardashian's stay while giving birth to her daughter.

To avoid such situations, celebrities often check into the hospital using aliases. However, Spears's own name was reportedly restored on her file when she left the hospital, apparently in an effort to keep her health information in one record. Other high-profile people, such as politicians, check in under aliases as well. Even so, employees at New York-Presbyterian Hospital allegedly tried to gain unauthorized access to Bill Clinton's health records when he had cardiac surgery in 2004. The records of crime victims whose names have been in the news also have been viewed improperly.

In all of these cases the hackers or would-be hackers are on the inside. They are people with legitimate access to the institution's computer system and perhaps to certain patients' records, but not to the records of the VIPs whose records they're trying to peek at. In 2008, a former employee of UCLA Medical Center was indicted for selling confidential health information in exchange for a mere $4,600. The hospital discovered that at least 31 celebrities' records had been accessed without authorization, and at least a dozen employees have been fired for letting curiosity or greed get the better of them. These breaches are prohibited by HIPAA, a law intended to protect the privacy of all patients in the United States. Civil and criminal penalties can be imposed for violating the law.

High-profile patients have just as much right to medical privacy as the rest of us, but why should we be concerned?

Every time another well-publicized privacy breach occurs, we lose a little more confidence that our own records are safe from prying eyes. According to a 2013 Health Information Trends Survey, 12.3% of us admit to having withheld information from our physicians for fear it will end up on TMZ someday—or at least in the hands of a nosy coworker, neighbor, or relative. This percentage is higher among those who are in worse health, and when our physicians don't have a complete picture of our health status, the care they're able to provide suffers.

The lack of widely available and interoperable electronic records, in turn, hampers public health surveillance of diseases such as cancer, hepatitis, and influenza. (Researchers are exempt from HIPAA and may access patients' health information as long their identities are kept confidential.) Such monitoring is important because it allows agencies like the CDC to spot patterns, such as an increase in the incidence of tuberculosis. It was just such public health surveillance that helped scientists recognize HIV/AIDS as a new disease in the early 1980s. If electronic records had been available then, it's likely the pattern would have emerged sooner, spurring prevention efforts and research into treatments.

In addition, researchers use EHR systems to find and recruit participants for clinical trials. For example, a researcher might search an EHR database to determine how many men ages 25 to 34 use chewing tobacco. The researcher can then ask each patient's physician to notify him that he is eligible for the study. An EHR system can even be customized so that when he visits his physician, every man in the correct age range is asked about his use of smokeless tobacco. Researchers can also cross-check chewing tobacco use against clinical data recorded in the EHR, such as blood pressure, to look for an association between tobacco use and high blood pressure.

These are just some of the ways in which EHR systems improve public health. For you as an individual patient, having an EHR promotes your health in a host of ways. For example, you're less likely to suffer an adverse drug reaction due to a drug dosage error when your provider is prescribing medications electronically. However, media hype about high-profile privacy violations tends to get us all wondering who might want to take a gander at our records—and that's bad news for everyone's health.

EARLY VERSUS LATE ADOPTERS

Most patients and members of the healthcare community agree that the advantages of EHR systems outweigh the disadvantages. Yet there are still a few paper pushers left in the field, holding on to their clipboards until the last moment. Of those who have implemented EHR systems, few use all the tools the system has to offer. The disadvantages outlined explain why many medical practices are hesitant to go digital, even with the pressures of government. So who *is* using EHR systems?

A large study showed that those most likely to have adopted EHR systems were primary care physicians, physicians practicing in large groups (in hospitals and medical centers), and specialists. In addition, recent healthcare graduates are among those who report overall satisfaction with EHR usage. These providers believe the systems can improve patients' quality of care, but they also noted the financial cost as the strongest barrier to implementation.

Since 2010, user satisfaction among healthcare providers has decreased a bit; providers cite inefficient EHR usability and lack of continuous training. So what characteristics can predict success and satisfaction with the system? A 2012 study of primary care physicians found that the following factors affect user satisfaction:

- Length of system response time
- Perception of whether workflow is logical and efficient
- Ability to complete desired tasks
- Ease of correcting mistakes
- Length of time required to learn and use the system
- Availability of proper training and support throughout the conversion process

- Perception of how the system affects quality of care
- Ability to convert to the system voluntarily, versus a mandatory conversion
- Level of prior computing skills

ROLE OF THE HEALTHCARE PROFESSIONAL USING THE ELECTRONIC HEALTH RECORD

The EHR has many users within the healthcare environment and will have an effect on all areas of the medical office. Physicians, nurses, physician's assistants, medical assistants, and medical coders and billers all must use or be exposed to the EHR. Although learning new software may be difficult and time consuming, it is important to keep patient care front and center at all times. Having certain basic skills can help you use an EHR effectively:

- **A working knowledge of medical terminology and anatomy and physiology.** The healthcare staff is responsible for documenting the patient's health history and status. Proper documentation of the patient's medical care is much easier for those who are familiar with medical terminology and have a solid grasp of how the body works. The EHR user also has to interpret information already documented in the patient chart, and many physicians use an alphabet soup of medical abbreviations. Therefore, the ability to decipher medical information will continue to be one of the main job duties of the healthcare staff.
- **Basic typing and computer skills.** Ventres and colleagues found that the ability to type was crucial to effective use of the EHR system. The providers in this study also noted that the ability to type is key to limiting transcription costs in their practices. Although free text writing is not the primary method of documentation within the patient medical record, some narrative data entry is required. The ability to type also eases navigation through the system.
- **Organizational skills.** The physician's office is busy and hectic most of the day. Patients are coming in and out of the office, the telephone is constantly ringing, and the stack of "to-do's" piles up on the desk. It's important for the healthcare staff to remain calm and properly manage their time and responsibilities. The EHR can help organize an office by keeping all of the patient data in one place, but it also takes time and grunt work to keep the records updated. Strong organizational skills are required to ensure patients' care and office workflow are managed effectively on busy days.
- **Interpersonal skills.** The genuine desire to work with people is a requirement for anyone in the medical field. The healthcare staff should always demonstrate a positive, warm, caring attitude toward their patients and coworkers. These skills include maintaining eye contact during communication, speaking slowly and clearly, and listening carefully. All staff members must show respect at all times during patient encounters and with one another. It is important to remember that converting to an EHR is a learning process for everyone, and not all individuals will catch on at the same time. Patience and a helpful personality are the key to keeping staff morale at its highest.

Duties and Workflow

The modern healthcare worker must possess basic skills and attributes when using the EHR. Many medical care facilities may require or prefer their employees to be cross-trained in various areas of the medical office. *Cross-training* means being able to perform more than one duty or skill across various task areas. Cross-training is especially helpful in a healthcare environment when a coworker calls in sick or is otherwise unable to perform his or her typical duties. Along with cross-training, the healthcare provider should be flexible and able to multitask. The implementation of new EHR software takes time and patience. The healthcare worker may become frustrated with the additional work and new way of performing daily tasks, but must remember to keep the patients' care the top priority.

Administrative

The adoption of an EHR system affects many of the administrative duties within the medical office. Medical office personnel will need to adapt to these changes to ensure a smooth transition from paper-based records to EHR systems. The EHR is purchased in a generic format and must be customized to fit a given office. Doing so represents a large chunk of the administrative work in a medical office. Some of the other administrative tasks include:

- Reception (front office) duties
- Appointment scheduling
- Electronic chart creation
- Inactive chart purging
- Gathering and entering patient information
- Creating patient correspondence
- Maintaining email communications
- Providing patient instructions
- Coordinating patient care (including setting up patient referrals, treatments, procedures)

Clinical

The EHR is a great way to coordinate a patient's care and document the record of treatment. The EHR can be customized to ensure that all components of the patient visit are well documented. As discussed, some of the clinical information that may be documented using the EHR includes patient history, vital signs, progress notes, laboratory requisitions, prescriptions, and test results.

Billing and Coding

Fully integrated EHR and practice management systems allow the user to review the clinical documentation while preparing claims for submission. Data from patient demographics and Superbill are populated into the insurance claim. The EHR aids in billing and coding tasks in the following ways:

- Submission of Superbills
- Creation of billing statements
- Assignment of procedural and diagnostic codes
- Linking of procedural and diagnostic codes for reimbursement
- Auditing
- Organizing office finance (day sheets, deposit slips, and patient account ledgers)
- Generating prior authorization forms
- Monitoring the submission and follow-up of claims (insurance claim tracers)

PROFESSIONAL ORGANIZATIONS

Learning should be lifelong, especially in a constantly changing environment like healthcare. Current healthcare trends, like International Classification of Diseases (ICD) 10 transition, EHR implementation, HIPAA policy, and patient engagement, are a main focus of professional organizations to help their members be skillfully competent in their job duties. Depending on your chosen field, you will want to become a member of one or more professional organizations. Many professional organizations offer discounted student memberships. All of the professional organizations listed here have one thing in common: They all aim to provide an up-to-date, informed approach to healthcare. These organizations have a wide variety of membership benefits, including the following:

- Offer certification exams at a discounted rate
- Provide a wide range of continuing education unit (CEU) opportunities
- Provide a forum for networking with other professionals in your field of study

- Publish newsletters and magazines dealing with current issues and trends in healthcare
- Offer discounts on publications
- Sponsor conferences, workshops, and web-based activities

With the advent of EHR systems, professional organizations are focusing on helping members adapt to the new technology and on research regarding its implementation in their medical offices. Professional publications, such as *Journal of AHIMA*, published by the American Health Information Management Association, *The Coding Edge*, published by the American Association of Professional Coders, and *CMA Today*, offered by the American Association of Medical Assistants (AAMA), regularly include articles and links related to the development and use and evaluation of EHR systems.

American Health Information Management Association

The American Health Information Management Association (AHIMA) is the leading professional organization made up of health information management (HIM) professionals. AHIMA has more than 71,000 members who are dedicated to the effective management of personal health information. Originally established in 1928 as the American Association of Record Librarians, AHIMA works to improve the quality of medical records for the diagnosis and treatment of health conditions. This professional organization is committed to advancing the HIM profession in critical topics such as privacy and security, medical coding, EHR systems, reimbursement, and compliance. AHIMA continues to develop new opportunities in an increasingly electronic and global environment through leadership in advocacy, education, certification, and lifelong learning. For more information, go to www.ahima.org.

American Academy of Professional Coders

The American Academy of Professional Coders (AAPC) was founded in 1988 in an effort to elevate the standards of medical coding by providing certification, ongoing education, networking, and recognition. The AAPC has a membership base of 126,000 worldwide. AAPC certifications focus on a variety of disciplines. These disciplines encompass the physician's office, represented by the Certified Professional Coder (CPC); the hospital outpatient facility, represented by the Certified Professional Coder–Hospital (CPC-H); and payer perspective coding, represented by the Certified Professional Coder–Payer (CPC-P). Specialty credentials are offered in evaluation and management, auditing, general surgery, obstetrics and gynecology, emergency medicine, and cardiology. The AAPC offers continuing education through local chapters, workshops, a monthly newsmagazine *(The Coding Edge)*, publications, and conferences. More information can be found at www.aapc.com.

American Association of Medical Assistants

The American Association of Medical Assistants (AAMA) is a professional organization for medical assistants searching for professional development, continuing education, approved programs, and certification information for medical assistants. The AAMA is vital to the accreditation process of medical assistant training programs and publishes a bimonthly journal called *CMA Today*. As far back as 2007, the Occupational Analysis of the CMA AAMA identified the use of computers and electronic equipment in the medical office as one of its key competencies. This skill is only becoming more and more important. You can further search the AAMA at www.aama-ntl.org.

American Medical Technologists

The American Medical Technologists (AMT) is a nonprofit certification agency and professional membership association representing more than 60,000 individuals in allied healthcare. Established in 1939, AMT provides allied health professionals with professional certification services and membership programs to enhance their professional and personal growth. The AMT publishes *AMT Events,* a quarterly magazine offering educational articles and professional development opportunities. For more information regarding the registered medical technologist, go to www.americanmedtech.org.

CHAPTER SUMMARY

- Patient health records have been used as early as 200 BCE to document treatment of patients and record signs and symptoms of illness. These records serve as important tools for research and have been traditionally paper-based records. Emerging technology is moving these documents into a digital form.
- The patient health record is a collection of an individual's healthcare information. It includes both patient information (demographics and insurance information) and clinical data (immunization records, operative reports, office notes, and so on). In addition, the patient medical record can be an important resource in legal actions and financial reimbursement matters. Attention must be paid to ensure the patient medical record is accurately maintained by all healthcare staff.
- Documentation is the process of recording data about a patient's health history and status or the chronologic record that results from such data entry. Taken together, it is a legal document and a key component of an EHR. Documentation may include clinical observations and progress notes, diagnoses of illnesses and injuries, plans of care, patient education and self-care instructions given, vital signs taken, physical assessment findings, laboratory and imaging test results, medical treatments prescribed or administered, surgeries performed, and outcomes.
- The patient medical record or patient chart is the property of its creator. For example, if a physician's office creates the patient medical record, the record itself is the property of the physician's office. Control of the information within the medical record belongs to the patient. A patient may request a copy of his or her medical record or view its contents by signing a release.
- The IOM has developed a list of eight core standards that every EHR should meet. These are health information and data management, results management, order management, decision support, electronic communication and connectivity, patient support, administration processes, and reporting and population health.
- Basic functions of EHR software include documentation using electronic transcription, provider review of incoming lab data and reports, electronic prescribing, transcription, and automatically generated clinical flags and reminders. Clinical decision support is an advanced feature of EHR software. This function comprises a set of tools that can improve patient safety, ensure that care conforms to established clinical guidelines for specific conditions, and reduce unnecessary care, duplicated services, and their associated costs.
- Practice management software is used for administrative duties in the medical office and is commonly an integrated part of the EHR. It can be used to enter patient demographics and insurance information, schedule appointments, and perform advanced accounting functions.
- The advantages of using an EHR system include improved quality and continuity of care, increased efficiency, improved documentation, easier point-of-care accessibility, better security, reduced expenses, improved job satisfaction for providers and staff, and improved patient satisfaction.
- The disadvantages of using an EHR system include lack of interoperability, a high cost of initial investment in time and money, resistance from some employees, regimentation as a result of using standardized templates to document patient care, and security gaps attributable to the electronic availability of confidential patient information.
- Factors such as length of response time and ease of correcting mistakes influence a practice's adoption of EHR systems.

- The roles of healthcare professionals change with the implementation of the EHR. Administrative, coding, billing, and clinical duties must all be refined to ensure a smooth transition from paper-based to electronic records systems.
- Membership and active involvement in professional organizations promote the use of EHR systems and broaden opportunities for valuable continuing education.

CHAPTER REVIEW ACTIVITIES

Key Terms Review

Match the following key terms with their definitions.

1. CPOE
2. Electronic transcription
3. Copayment
4. Interoperability
5. Ledger
6. Chief complaint
7. Reporting and population health
8. HIPAA 5010
9. Day sheet

a. The ability of electronic systems to share information in compatible formats

b. The patient's stated primary reason for seeking treatment

c. Screen that contains the amount owed and other billing details

d. An EHR function that facilitates automated prescribing

e. A fixed sum of money usually paid at the time medical services are rendered

f. An electronic format that speeds the claims process for physicians and suppliers

g. A register of business transactions for a single day

h. Data entry using structured data entry or voice recognition

i. One of the eight core functions of an EHR designated by the IOM

True/False

Indicate whether the statement is true or false.

1. _____ An audit is performed by the office manager to investigate whether appropriate employees have viewed the contents of a high-profile patient's chart.
2. _____ The medical record contains legal documents but is not itself a legal document.
3. _____ The medical assistant's typical duties will be modified with the implementation of the EHR.
4. _____ Clinical decision support tools are effective only if the provider chooses to use them.
5. _____ An EHR system can help the provider and medical staff plan and coordinate care for a patient with a chronic illness.
6. _____ Automated sentence building is a means of electronic transcription.
7. _____ Reduced productivity is to be expected for a period of time during the conversion to an EHR system.
8. _____ Communication among various treating healthcare providers, pharmacies, and allied healthcare workers will be limited until EHR interoperability has been achieved.
9. _____ One of the core functions of the EHR includes the ability to assist providers with treatment protocols.
10. _____ It is possible for individuals to penetrate EHR systems despite security precautions.
11. _____ EHR systems make it unnecessary for office staff to be familiar with medical terminology.
12. _____ Most EHR systems hold the ability to handle clinical and administrative functions without purchasing separate practice management software.
13. _____ Professional organizations offer continuing education for the core skills of their discipline and do not have any opportunities for learning about the EHR.

Workplace Applications

1. Jamie is considering becoming a member of a professional organization but is unsure of the benefits. He's a new medical assistant in a practice with five physicians, and he hopes to become the office manager at a larger practice someday. To which professional organization should Jamie belong? What services does this organization provide that will help Jamie achieve his goals?

2. Kathy works for a pediatrician's office that is beginning the EHR implementation process. She has been asked to research the different systems available and general start-up cost. Create a list of functions the EHR should have specific to the practice's large pediatric office. What are the general start-up costs of EHR systems?

3. During an EHR training session you are leading for staff, one of the members states that she is upset with the new EHR requirements and the changes to her job duties. How can you ease her fears and help her understand the need for EHRs?

BIBLIOGRAPHY

Burke, L., & Weill, B. (2009). *Information technology for the health professions* (3rd ed.). Upper Saddle River, NJ: Pearson.

Chadwick-Dias, A. C., McNulty, M., & Tullis, T. *Web usability and age: An update.* Fidelity Investments: Fidelity Center for Applied Technology, Human Interface Design. Available at http://hid.fidelity.com/q32002/age.htm. Accessed 03.12.08.

The Commonwealth Fund Commission on a High Performance Health System. (2007). *A high performance health system for the United States: An ambitious agenda for the next president.* Available at www.commonwealthfund.org/usr_doc/Ambitious_Agenda_1075.pdf?section=4039. Accessed 03.12.08.

DesRoches, C., Campbell, E. G., Sowmya, R. R., et al. (2008). Electronic health records in ambulatory care: A national survey of physicians. *New England Journal of Medicine*, 359, 50–60.

Employee Benefits Research Institute. (2008). Health confidence survey. *EBRI Notes.* Available at www.ebri.org/pdf/notespdf/EBRI_Notes_10-2008.pdf. Accessed 02.12.08.

Fordney, M. T. (2012). *Insurance handbook for the medical office* (12th ed.). St. Louis: Mosby.

Johnson, K. B., Serwint, J. R., & Fagan, L. A. (2008). Computer-based documentation: Effects on parent-provider communication during pediatric health maintenance encounters. *Pediatrics*, 122, 3.

Koppel, R., Metlay, J. P., Cohen, A., et al. (2005). Role of computerized physician order entry systems in facilitating medication errors. *Journal of the American Medical Association*, 293, 1197–1203. Available at http://jama.ama-assn.org/cgi/content/full/293/10/1197. Accessed 04.12.08.

MedChi: The Maryland State Medical Society Law and Advocacy Division. (2008). *Update on medical records copying charges.* Sept. 10. www.medchi.orgs/lawandadvocacy/MedRec_Fees.asp. Accessed 04.12.08.

Miller, R. H., West, C., Brown, T. M., et al. (2005). The value of electronic health records in solo or small group practices. *Health Affairs (Millwood)*, 24, 1127–1137.

National Center for Health Statistics, Centers for Disease Control and Prevention. *National health care surveys information sheet.* Available at www.cdc.gov/nchs/data/infosheets/infosheet_nhcs.htm. Accessed 02.12.08.

Pew Research Center. (2008). *Networked workers.* Sept 24. Pew Internet and American Life Project. Available at http://pewresearch.org/pubs/966/networked-workers. Accessed 04.12.08.

Trachtenberg, D. E. (2007). EHRs fix everything—and nine other myths. *Family Practice Management*, 14(3):26–30.

Ventres, W., Kooienga, S., Vuckovic, N., et al. (2006). Physicians, patients, and the electronic health record: An ethnographic analysis. *Annals of Family Medicine*, 4, 124–131.

Young, A., & Proctor, D. (2011). *Kinn's the medical assistant: An applied learning approach* (11th ed.). St. Louis: Mosby.

chapter 2

Overview of SimChart for the Medical Office

Chapter Outline

Commission on Accreditation of Allied Health Education Programs (CAAHEP) Competencies

1. Discuss principles of using electronic medical records (EMRs).
2. Use the Internet to access information related to the medical office.
3. Use office hardware and software to maintain office systems.
4. Execute data management using electronic healthcare records such as the EMR.

Chapter Objectives

1. Describe the medical assistant's role in promoting electronic health records.
2. Log in to SCMO.
3. Find and use the Student Resources available for SCMO.
4. Understand how to view and submit assignments in SCMO.
5. Access the SCMO Simulation Playground and navigate across modules.
6. Identify common buttons and other recurrent elements in SCMO.
7. Explain the difference between active and closed records.
8. Create new patient records in SCMO.
9. Discuss the appropriate use of the Internet in the physician's office.

Key Terms

active patient   An established patient who has seen the provider or another provider in the billing group within the past 3 years.

button   An element of the user interface on which the user can click to execute a command, such as confirm, cancel, or exit.

check box   A specialized type of button that toggles on (checked) and off (unchecked). Check boxes are often used when more than one response might be appropriate (as in "Check all that apply"), but sometimes they should be interpreted to mean yes or no (as in a check box next to the caption "OK to mail?").

closed patient record   The record of a patient who has not been seen by the provider or any other provider in the billing group in 3 or more years.

default   A preselected value or setting that will be used unless the user specifies a substitute by overriding the preselected choice.

field   Space allocated on a form for specific numeric or text data.

radio button   A specialized type of button on a software interface that toggles on (round button visible) and off (blank circle). Radio buttons tell the user that only one response is appropriate because two radio buttons can't be depressed at the same time.

retention period   The amount of time patient records must, by law, be maintained by the medical office.

THE MEDICAL PRACTICE GOES DIGITAL

According to the U.S. Department of Labor, electronic health record (EHR) systems are good for business—at least when it comes to medical assisting. As standards of interoperability have been adopted and financial incentives for EHR use have become more attractive, adoption of EHR systems has reached a tipping point. This circumstance has made medical assisting one of the fastest-growing professions in the United States.

According to the 2013 Medical Assisting Compensation and Benefits Report of 4400 respondents, 64% of medical assistants work in primary care practice. Another 32% work with medical or surgical specialty offices, 2.6% report employment in emergency and outpatient hospital departments, and 1.1% work in ambulatory surgery centers. Only 7% of survey responders selected "Other" as employment type. Tech-savvy medical assistants are in great demand, often commanding higher salaries and landing positions in the most desirable practices.

The EHR has been slow to take root in physicians' offices, but healthcare personnel have come to appreciate its potential to streamline office management and improve patient care. A comprehensive EHR can be used to schedule patients, establish and maintain health records, ensure continuity of care, improve communication, document clinical work, and perform billing and coding functions. The remaining transition will take years or perhaps even a generation, but many practices are eager to catch up, and medical assistants continue to stand at the forefront of this digital transition. If you're just getting your feet wet, don't worry—you have plenty of time to learn. The Glossary for Computer Novices located at the end of this chapter is a great place to start.

In this chapter we put the top down and take the EHR out for a spin. Although you'll be using SimChart for the Medical Office (SCMO), you won't be wasting your time if you end up working in an office that uses a different software application. Using SCMO is sort of like familiarizing yourself with the controls of a vehicle—once you have that experience under your belt, you will feel comfortable behind the wheel of any car.

SCMO simulates the real-life application of the EHR. It is a primary care office with three providers: Dr. James A. Martin, Dr. Julie Walden, and nurse practitioner Jean Burke. You will also get to know a variety of the office's existing patients like sweet Norma Washington, independent Celia Tapia, and accountant Al Neviaser, just to name a few. You can also add new patients, which we will do a little later in this chapter.

EASING THE TRANSITION 2-1

Digital Basics for Computer Novices

Today, there's a PC in every cubicle and a mobile device in every hand. You can download an "app" for any game, food diary, or pregnancy predictor (just to name a few) you desire. Information is at our fingertips, and patients expect their physician's office to be just as connected. After all, healthcare is also one of the most high-tech businesses in America. But EHR adoption is still low. Regardless of their age, healthcare personnel have often skated around computer use by working in clinical settings. It may take a generation, says John Hsu, an anesthesiologist who has written about the problem, before computer-phobic healthcare personnel are replaced by more tech-savvy workers. And therein lies a key factor—the human factor—in resistance to EHR adoption, says Hsu.

Invariably, some staff members will plead computer illiteracy and expect to be let off the hook when an EHR is introduced to the practice. A physician may want to retain his own paper files, or a longtime staff member might somehow expect to float outside the system—take vitals, say, and let someone else enter them into the EHR. But allowing parallel paper and electronic systems to exist beyond the transitional period is like having one person in a design studio creating illustrations on mat boards while the other six graphic artists use Photoshop.

Compromise may be a good thing, but it's not what's needed when a clinician or staffer tries to opt out of converting to the EHR. Strong leadership and a heavy dose of enthusiasm will generally carry the day. Owen O'Neill, a champion of his practice's EHR, was both delighted and astonished to watch physicians in his group with only rudimentary computer skills become versatile EHR users. These computer converts tend to take advantage of more of the EHR's features, O'Neill notes, perhaps because they participated in additional training. With that in mind, be sure everyone on your staff is familiar with the computing terms and concepts outlined in Table 2-2. After all, you don't want to end up a PEBCAK—that's geek speak for "Problem Exists Between Chair And Keyboard."

CRITICAL THINKING EXERCISE 2-1

Consider your own experience with medical office technology. If you've had experience using an electronic appointment book or a full-blown EHR, how has it helped you and your patients? If you haven't, think about other ways in which technology has been useful to you—in school, for example, or in a job outside the medical field. How do you think a person's attitude toward technology influences that of the people they work with?

CRITICAL THINKING EXERCISE 2-2

Review the Glossary for Computer Novices, located at the end of this chapter. Which computer terms are new to you? How would the computer concepts apply to the medical setting? Other than EHRs, in what type of scenarios could you use the computer to enhance patient care?

ACCESSING SCMO THROUGH EVOLVE

1. From the main menu of your computer, open Mozilla Firefox. (Evolve and SCMO are compatible with most browsers, but Chrome or Mozilla Firefox works best.)
2. Go to http://evolve.elsevier.com/enroll.
3. Under Step 2 on the page, click on the link to self-enroll.
4. Enter the course ID in the field (provided by your instructor) and click Submit (Figure 2-1).

Figure 2-1
Evolve Course Enroll-
ment screen.

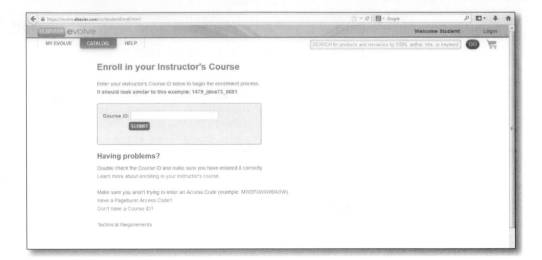

5. A pop up window asking you to log in or create a new account will appear. If you are a returning user, enter your Evolve username and password and click Login. If you are new to Evolve, enter your name, email, desired password, institution information (if applicable) and click Continue.

6. If you have a 12-character access code, type it into the field provided and select Apply. Note: Access codes may only be used once. If you do not have an access code, SimChart for the Medical Office is available for purchase.

7. Next, select Redeem/Checkout. (Note: You may be prompted to update your account information at this point. Ensure it is still accurate before continuing.)

8. Check the box to accept the Registered User Agreement.

9. Click Submit

10. Your enrollment confirmation will appear on the next page. A confirmation email will additionally be sent to your instructor to inform him or her of your enrollment. If you are a new user, your Evolve username and password will also be emailed to you.

11. Click the Get Started link to get to your course located in the My Evolve area. Visit and bookmark http://evolve.elsevier.com/student for future logins.

GETTING COMFORTABLE WITH ELECTRONIC HEALTH RECORDS SOFTWARE

SCMO is a type of software as a service (SAAS). SCMO is able to function in a variety of locations, such as a medical office, classroom, lab, home—basically anywhere you have Internet access. The EHR system includes Front Office, Clinical Care, and Coding and Billing modules to provide real-life application in a safe learning environment. All users have their own access into the system, so you do not need to worry about any of your work showing up on someone else's screen. All of your data is specific to you, so feel free to explore. This includes spending time looking around, becoming familiar with the available resources, and examining the EHR functions and tools of the Simulation Playground. As with any new skill, practice makes perfect.

Resources for SCMO

SCMO has a robust number of resources to help you get the most from the system. You can access these from the Evolve page. The link for Student Resources is found on the left side info panel, listed under Course Content (Figure 2-2).

Here's a summary of some of the items you will find listed in SCMO Student Resources: Getting Started:

- Quick Tips for Students
- Modules

Figure 2-2
Student Resources link.

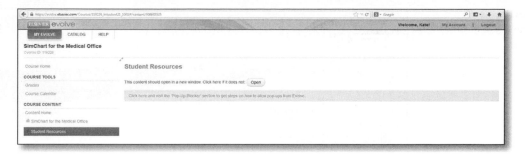

- Simulation Playground
- Student FAQ
- Glossary
- Info Panel Guide
- Getting Starting
- Assignments
  - Assignments Overview
  - Completing and Submitting Assignments
  - Reattempting Assignments
- Grading
  - Grading Overview
  - Reviewing Graded Assignments
- Job Readiness
  - Student Portfolio Tips
  - Job Readiness Skills
  - Becoming a Successful MA Student
  - SCMO as a Marketable Asset

SCMO ASSIGNMENT VIEW

When you enter SCMO from the Evolve portal, you will be directed to the Assignment page. From this page you can access the EHR Simulation Playground. This is a practice environment that allows you to explore a fully functioning EHR and familiarize yourself with the features and workflows available. As within the rest of the system, you can save work, print, return to previous entries, and build patients all in this practice setting.

The Open Assignments grid within the Assignment page (Figure 2-3) displays assignments released by your instructor. This grid displays the assignment title, module, estimated duration, and status of an assignment. Once you click on the assignment title, you will enter the assignment portal, which contains:

- Description: An EHR case study with listed objectives and attachments
- Competencies: A list of any accreditation competencies covered in the assignment
- Quiz: A series of content questions related to the assignment. The assignment cannot be submitted until the quiz is complete.
- Additional Resources

You can toggle back and forth between these sections but must click the Start Assignment button in the bottom right corner of the Description section to start the simulation portion of an assignment. The Front Office calendar is the default landing page for all assignments. From this view you must use the details in the Assignment Description to determine how to complete the tasks in an assignment. There is a View Assignment Description in the top right corner just in case you forget any assignment details. The assignment title displays at the top of the screen in black text, distinguishing this environment from the regular Playground environment. Once you complete your EHR activity, click the Back to Assignment link to the left of the View Assignment Description link in order to answer the quiz questions. These questions refer to simulation activity in some

Figure 2-3
Open Assignment table screen.

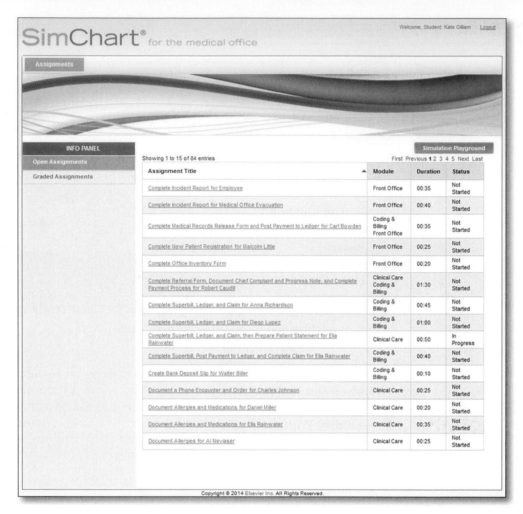

cases, but most questions address general best practices. Instructors manually evaluate student activity within the simulation portion of an assignment, but the system automatically grades answers to quiz questions and generates a preliminary score for the assignment. You can view your preliminary score within the Graded Assignments tab of the Info Panel. Once your instructor reviews your simulation work and approves this automatically generated score, the grade will become bold.

MODULES

SCMO is organized into three modules established to simulate the medical office workflow, following a patient visit from start to finish. Just think of the patient's experience in the medical office. Typically a patient enters the medical office, fills out paperwork, and is escorted into the examination room. After the initial intake procedures, the patient is examined by the physician, has procedures performed, and is billed for services. Keeping this workflow in mind, SCMO is organized into Front Office, Clinical Care, and Coding and Billing.

Front Office

As mentioned, the Front Office calendar is the default landing page of the simulation (Figure 2-4). The office staff views the calendar more frequently than most pages in order to effectively manage patient visits. Users can create, edit, and delete new or established patient appointments. An appointment matrix can be established by adding block or other

Figure 2-4
Front Office menus.

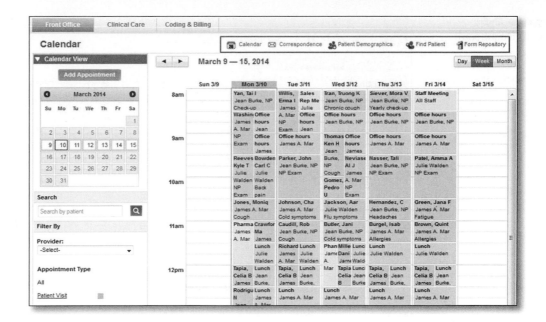

appointment slots such as staff meetings, lunch hours, or sales meetings. Other administrative functions within the Front Office module include composing patient letters, phone messages, and emails with the use of the Correspondence menu. The Patient Demographics tool is used to establish and manage patient and payer information. The Form Repository provides a comprehensive set of office forms. All of the documents and data created in the Front Office module can be viewed, saved to patient records, and printed. We will use the Front Office module in Chapter 5.

Clinical Care

View and document all patient care within the Clinical Care module, accessed by clicking the Clinical Care tab or the Find Patient icon. Once a patient is selected, SCMO will display a summary of all patient record entries known as the Patient Dashboard (Figure 2-5). In addition to viewing the contents of the patient's record, you can add a new encounter or enter an existing encounter. All clinical documentation is performed within a patient encounter. Users must be in a patient encounter before documenting any clinical care. This reminds us that clinical documentation is performed within a visit between a patient and healthcare provider. There are several clinical records for data entry:

- Allergies
- Chief Complaint
- Health History
- Immunizations
- Medications
- Order Entry
- Patient Education
- Preventive Services
- Problem List
- Progress Note
- Vitals Signs

In addition to these clinical functions, the user can upload diagnostic and lab results with the help of the Form Repository in the Front Office module. All of these forms such as the Lab Requisition, Neurological Status Exam, and School Physical are used in real medical offices. We will learn more about clinical documentation in Chapter 6.

Figure 2-5
Patient Dashboard.

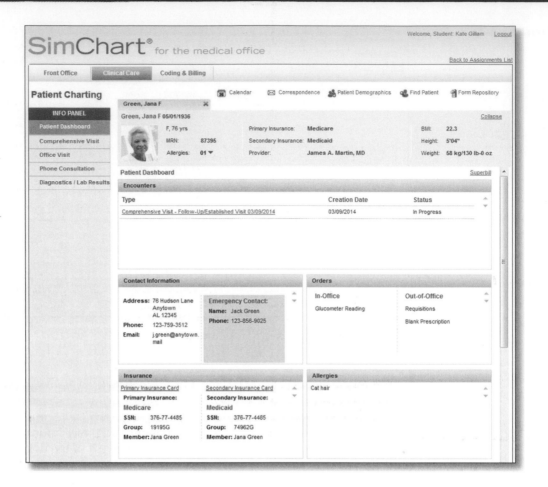

Coding and Billing

Considering all of the other documentation requirements and patient needs, it's easy to forget that a physician's office is a business. Managing the monies going in and out of the office is the primary responsibility of the billing and coding department and the focus of the last SCMO module. The main features of the Coding and Billing module include:

- Superbill
- Ledger
- Claim Processing
- Day Sheet

Just like the Front Office and Clinical Care, the Form Repository plays a large role in this module as well. Insurance specialists regularly use forms such as the Insurance Claim Tracer, Patient Statement, and Bank Deposit Slip. The user can practice coding skills and understand the importance of good documentation when reviewing the progress notes by completing the Superbill and claim. We look at the Coding and Billing module in greater detail in Chapter 7.

RECURRING FEATURES IN SCMO

As you move from screen to screen through SCMO, you will notice certain visual cues that indicate functionality. Many similar cues occur in other applications, so you may already be familiar with some of them. For instance, anyone who has ever made a purchase on eBay knows that a field marked in red on the billing and shipping form must be filled out before proceeding to the next screen. SCMO uses the same functionality.

Keyboard shortcuts, icons, dialog boxes, back buttons, forward arrows, drop-down menus, scroll bars, **check boxes,** and **radio buttons** are covered in the glossary at the end of the chapter. Many SCMO functions are content-specific, meaning that the tools and buttons available are specific to the task being performed. Let's look at a few elements and functions you will use repeatedly as you navigate through SCMO.

Buttons

The **buttons** in SCMO appear on nearly every module and screen. Some have graphics (for example, the green plus sign in immunizations) on them, and others have text labels (for example, the orange Add Appointment button in the Calendar). Most are activated by a single mouse click rather than a double click. When they appear in full color, they are active, or clickable. When the color of the button is faded or "grayed" out, it is a visual cue that they are inactive and can't be selected.

Default Settings

Many students first learn about **default** settings while preparing a term paper. Perhaps you were asked to use the margin widths specified in a particular style guide. Or maybe it was 11 PM and you were looking for a quick way to turn an 11-page paper into the required 15 pages. In either case, you would have had to override the margins already set for your document. Likewise, when you open a dialog box or screen in SCMO, the options you are most likely to select have already been chosen for you. These are called default options.

Info Panel

The SCMO Info Panel is located on the left side of the screen and changes depending on the module. The Info Panel in the Clinical Care setting is used to create an encounter or enter lab and diagnostic test results (Figure 2-6). The Coding and Billing module uses the Info Panel to toggle between the various responsibilities of a reimbursement specialist. Info Panels are also used in the Form Repository and Correspondence menu to indicate what templates are available in each tool.

Figure 2-6
Clinical Care Info panel.

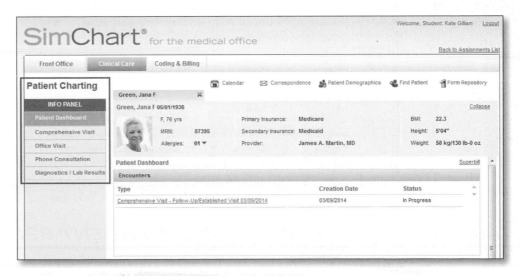

Structured and Unstructured Data Entry Options

There are a number of ways to enter data into electronic health record systems. The best thing you can do is get as much experience as possible in as many ways as possible.

Some EHR systems allow the user to use voice dictation or enter free-text data into text fields. This type of narrative is called unstructured data entry, and it allows flexibility in the physician's communications, observations, orders, and patient cases. For many physicians just starting to use an EHR system, this type of documentation is the most similar to that of paper records. It allows for a complete narrative picture of the physician's thoughts and easily illustrates a complete picture of the patient's case. Structured data entry uses coded data in several databases. The user identifies preexisting data from drop-down boxes, default settings, templates, and check boxes to document individual patient information. Structured data are easier to collect and share among other computer systems, which will aid system-wide interoperability. At first it seems like a quicker method of documentation because the data are already "typed" in for the user, but many physicians complain that this type of data entry takes longer to find a particular message. In addition, no one database can possibly contain all of the options a patient will present with, leading to significant limitations and loss of important data. SCMO gives the user experience in both types of data entry to best prepare medical assistants for the vast number of EHR systems they might encounter during an externship and on the job. For example, patient medications can be entered using a database of drugs or manually.

Find Patient Tool

You can imagine how time consuming and overwhelming it would be to scroll through lists and patient names to locate a particular patient. The Find Patient tool makes this task painless. When you type the first few letters of a patient's last name into the Last Name field and click the Go button, the EHR automatically displays matching items at the top of the list (Figure 2-7).

Figure 2-7
Find Patient tool.

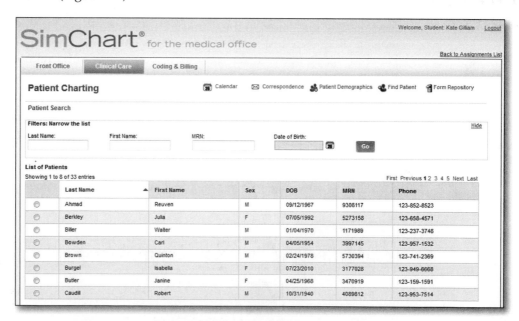

ESTABLISHING AND MAINTAINING A PATIENT REGISTRY

Active patients are established patients who currently see a physician or any healthcare provider in the group. **Closed patient records** are those of patients who have not been seen in the past 3 years. Only registered, active patients can be scheduled for appointments. This group of active patients is called the *patient registry* or *master patient index*. Active patient health records are maintained, and closed patient records are purged from the EHR as soon as it is legally advisable to do so. Closed patient records are placed into electronic storage, where they must be kept for liability reasons in the event of a medical malpractice suit. The **retention period** is the amount of time records must be kept (retained) in storage by a medical office. Table 2-1 shows the recommended retention time for paper files. Retention time for EHR systems is specified by law and varies from state to state. SCMO has about 30 preloaded active patients in the master patient index, but you can use the Add Patient button anytime to create more patients. Let's show you how next!

CRITICAL THINKING EXERCISE 2-3

Give some other examples of technologic skills that are transferable from one version or model of an EHR product to another.

Table 2-1   Records Retention Schedule

Temporary Record	Retention Period (Years)	Permanent Record (Retained Indefinitely)
Accounts receivable (patient ledger)	7	
Appointment sheets	3	Accounts payable records
Bank deposit slips (duplicate)	1	Bills of sale for important purchases (or until you no longer own them); canceled checks and check registers
Bank statements and canceled checks	7	Capital asset records
		Cash books
Billing records (for outside service)	7	Certified financial statements
Cash receipt records	6	Contracts
		Correspondence, legal
Contracts (expired)	7	Credit history
Correspondence, general	6	Deeds, mortgages, contracts, leases, and property records
Day sheets (balance sheets and journals)	5	Equipment guarantees and records (or until you no longer own them)
Employee contracts	6	Income tax returns and documents
Employee time records	5	Insurance policies and records
Employment applications	4	Journals (financial)
Insurance claim forms (paid)	3	
Inventory records	3	
Invoices	6	Health records (active patients)
Health records (expired patients)	5	Health records (inactive patients)
Medicare financial records	7	
Remittance advice documents	8	Mortgages
Payroll records	7	Property appraisals and records
Petty cash vouchers	3	Telephone records
Postal and meter records	1	X-ray films
Tax worksheets and supporting documents	7	Year-end balance sheets and general ledgers

From Fordney, M. T. (2008). *Insurance handbook for the medical office* (10th ed.). St. Louis: Saunders.

CRITICAL THINKING EXERCISE 2-4

Donna is new to your physician's office. While training her on the office EHR, she asks why closed patient records have to be retained. What qualifies as a closed record, and why must the record be placed in storage?

Enter a New Patient in SCMO

Now that you have successfully entered the EHR, it's time to see what it can do. Let's start by registering a new patient. Remember that we will be working in the Simulation Playground for this activity. As you follow along, try to register yourself as a "mock" patient.

1. From the Assignment page, click the Simulation Playground button located in the top right corner.
2. Select the top radio button to enter the Playground with all of the saved information from your previous session (Figure 2-8).

Figure 2-8
Playground confirmation box.

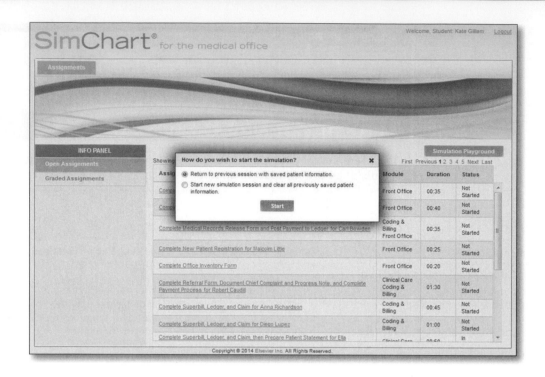

3. Click the Patient Demographics icon (Figure 2-9).

Figure 2-9
Patient Demographics tool.

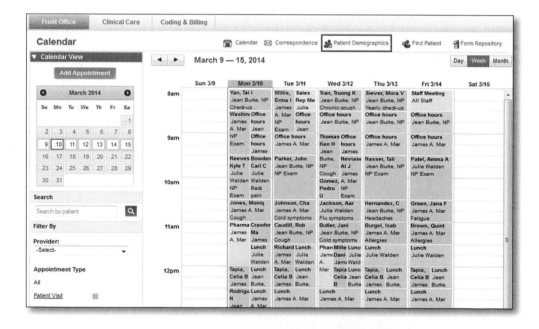

4. Attempt a patient search by entering the first couple of letters of the patient's last name in the Last Name field. Click the Search Existing Patients button (Figure 2-10).
5. If no patient record exists, the Add Patient button will appear under the search field. Click on the Add Patient button to create a new record (Figure 2-11).
6. The Patient Demographics–Add Patient window appears, organized using Patient, Guarantor, and Insurance tabs (Figure 2-12). Start by entering the Patient information, including name (as it appears on the insurance card or ID). The medical record number is automatically generated for the account, so there is no need to create one.
7. Complete the required fields within the Patient, Guarantor, and Insurance tabs. Red asterisks indicate required fields. New data entry is always required when a new billing account is created.

Figure 2-10
Patient Demographics
search field.

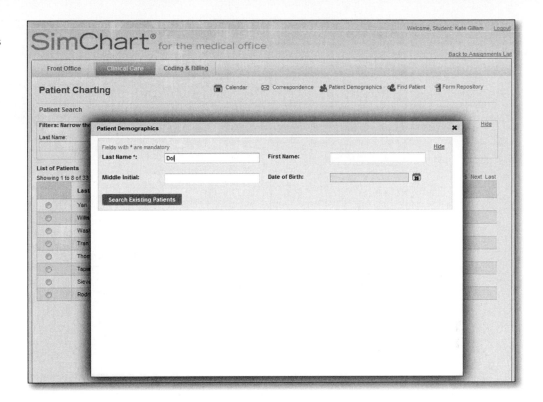

Figure 2-11
Patient Demographics
data screen.

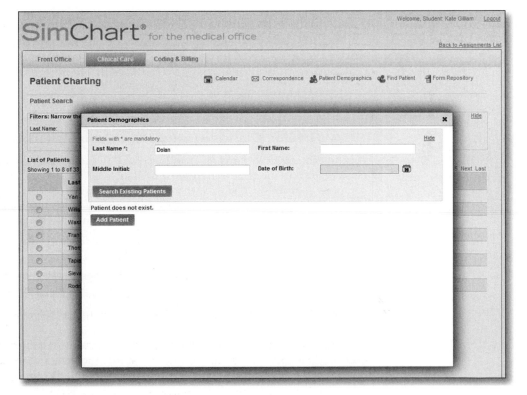

8. If a patient is self-insured, the user can select the Self radio button in the Guarantor tab and the patient information will auto-feed from the Patient tab. If the user selects an existing guarantor, that person's data will auto-populate into the fields.

9. The Insurance tab records Primary and Secondary Insurance Carriers. A scanned image of the insurance card can be attached to the account using the Upload Insurance Card link.

Figure 2-12
Patient Demographics
Add Patient button.

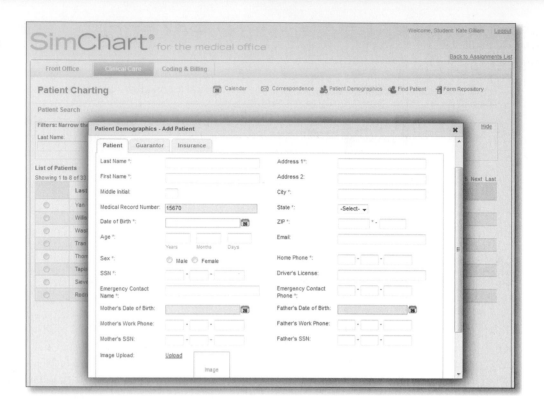

10. Scroll to the bottom of the Patient Demographics window and click the Save Patient button to create your new patient record. Your new patient is now part of the patient list.

As patient information changes, the Patient Demographics data can be updated as well.

EHR EXERCISE 2-1:   CREATE A NEW PATIENT RECORD

*Using the previous steps as a guide, complete the following exercise in the EHR Exercises environment of SimChart for the Medical Office.

Now that we have walked through how to register a new patient, let's see if you can establish a new patient record for Susannah Ling. Susannah is a new patient of Dr. Martin. Use the completed Patient Information form (located at the end of this chapter) to abstract and enter her data.

EHR EXERCISE 2-2:   EDIT PATIENT DEMOGRAPHICS

*Using the previous steps as a guide, complete the following exercise in the EHR Exercises environment of SimChart for the Medical Office.

Monique Jones, an established patient of Dr. Martin, stopped in the office this morning because the group number of her insurance has changed. Her Blue Cross/Blue Shield group number is now 78452K. Update Monique's demographics.

EHR EXERCISE 2-3:   CREATE A NEW PATIENT RECORD

*Using the previous steps as a guide, complete the following exercise in the EHR Exercises environment of SimChart for the Medical Office.

Two new patients, Chase Murray and Miles Green, are establishing with Dr. Walden today. Use the completed Patient Information forms (located at the end of the chapter) to create the new patient records.

INTERNET USE IN THE MEDICAL PRACTICE

Professional Use

The Internet is a great resource for the medical office. For SCMO, it is a necessary tool for access. In addition, members of the healthcare team may use it to locate testing centers for patients, identify appropriate clinical trials, find links to community support groups, and print patient education material. However, you should surf with caution. Although many reliable sites exist, many more offer bogus advice, usually in an effort to sell a useless or even harmful product or service. Patients and staff should be sure to determine what the agenda of the site is and whether the information at the URL is reliable. (See the Glossary for Computer Novices for an explanation of the terms *link* or *hyperlink, website* or *web page,* and *URL.*)

Personal Use

Of course, the Internet also has infinite personal uses—reading a favorite blog (or writing one), checking out friends' Facebook or Twitter status, swapping photos on Instagram, and maybe shopping for a fierce pair of Italian leather pumps from Zappos. There are more mundane uses for the Internet, too. In a spare moment you may find yourself trying to obtain the new level of Candy Crush, wandering over to see whether your check has cleared, paying your cell phone bill, or looking for a new apartment before your lease is up. It should go without saying that none of these activities is acceptable in the medical office. It may be tempting, but you should confine personal web browsing and mobile device usage to your own time, using computers unconnected with your place of employment. (See Table 2-2 the Glossary for Computer Novices at the end of the chapter for a discussion of the term *browser.*)

Here are some sensible guidelines for Internet use in the medical office:

- Internet use should be limited to sites related to your job duties. Your Internet usage may be monitored by your employer.
- Do not use the computer to send or receive personal email messages.
- Do not open email messages, especially attachments, from unfamiliar senders.
- Perform a virus check daily. Many software programs do this for you automatically, but the programs must be kept up to date, usually by purchasing periodic upgrades.
- Be careful not to copy documents or images in violation of copyright laws.
  - Do not download any software or apps to an office PC without permission.

CHAPTER SUMMARY

- A rapidly increasing rate of EHR adoption has combined with multiskilled staff members to make medical assisting one of the fastest-growing professions in the United States.
  - Users will enroll in SCMO from the Evolve website with an access code.
  - There are a variety of Student Resources available for SCMO in Evolve.
  - The Assignments view is the access location for the Simulation Playground and Open and Graded Assignments.
  - SCMO simulates a primary care office with three providers: Dr. Martin, Dr. Walden, and Jean Burke, NP.
- The functionality and navigational features in SCMO overlap with those of similar EHR products. Some common elements of SCMO include buttons, default settings, info panels, structured data entry, and patient search.
- A new patient record can be created by clicking the Patient Demographics icon and searching by last name. Once you have confirmed that the patient does not already exist in the system, click the Add Patient button at the bottom of the search field.
- In the medical office, the Internet should be used only for tasks related to one's job. A member of the medical office staff might use the Internet to locate testing centers for patients, find information about support groups in the community, or print patient education materials. Caution must be taken to ensure that reliable, professional sites are consulted.

CHAPTER REVIEW ACTIVITIES

Key Terms Review

Match the following key terms with their definitions.

1. Radio button
2. Field
3. Check box
4. retention period
5. active patient

a. The amount of time records must be kept in storage by a medical office
b. A specialized graphic element that toggles on and off and is used when more than one option is correct
c. A specialized graphic element that toggles on and off and is used when only one response is appropriate because two of these buttons can't be depressed at the same time
d. Space allocated on a form for specific numeric or text data
e. Used to describe an established patient who currently sees the physician

SCMO Scavenger Hunt

Log into Evolve and find the answers to the following questions.

1. The website to log into Evolve is:_____
2. According to the Quick Tips resource, the landing page for the student is called: _____
3. Name four functions of the Front Office module:
4. SCMO has three healthcare providers. What is the first name of the nurse practitioner?
5. Name the date of birth for Norma Washington.
6. What tests are included in a TORCH panel (hint: blood test order)?
7. Name two insurance and billing documents found in the Form Repository.
8. Name the three types of correspondence generated by SCMO.
9. List the HPI elements identified in a chief complaint.
10. Who is the guarantor for patient Celia Tapia?

True/False

Indicate whether the statement is true or false.

1. _____ Most medical assistants are employed in inpatient settings.
2. _____ SCMO does not include the ability to create patient letters because it is easier to store these documents outside of the patient record.
3. _____ Unfortunately no two systems are the same, so knowing how to use one EHR will be little help in learning to use another.
4. _____ SCMO is used to document clinical data and does not function as a practice management software (PMS) system.
5. _____ The user must first perform a patient search before entering a new patient record.
6. _____ When creating a new patient account, the user must randomly select a number to be the medical record number.
7. _____ SCMO allows the user to enter up to three insurance carriers.
8. _____ To submit an assignment the user should perform the EHR activity and answer quiz questions.
9. _____ Another name for a Patient Registry is a *master patient index*.
10. _____ Closed patient records are the records of patients who have not been seen in the past 6 months.
11. _____ The New Patient screen contains a patient's contact information and demographics.
12. _____ Information from the Internet is not reliable enough to use for patient education.

Workplace Applications

Using the knowledge you obtained from the chapter, provide answers to the following cases.

1. You notice that the employees in your office have been spending company time using the Internet for personal use—primarily reading blogs, exchanging emails with friends, downloading music, and watching YouTube videos. Create an office policy for the employee handbook that prohibits the misuse of the Internet and describes in what situations it may be used.

2. Kara is new to your office and is slowly becoming familiar with the EHR. She has asked you to review some of the common elements and features in SCMO. Explore and then describe some uses to her.

PATIENT INFORMATION (Please use full legal name.)

Last Name:	Ling	Address 1:	234 Capeside Dr
First Name:	Susannah	Address 2:	--
Middle Initial:	--	City:	Anytown
Medical Record Number:	--	State:	AL
Date of Birth:	01/02/1973	Zip:	12345
Age:	43	Email:	susannah.ling@scmo.edu
Sex:	Female	Home Phone:	445-555-7897
SSN:	111-22-3333	Driver's License:	CA54841
Emergency Contact Name:	Yolanda Arnold	Emergency Contact Phone:	445-555-8525

GUARANTOR INFORMATION (Please use full legal name.)

Relationship of Guarantor to Patient:	Self		
Guarantor/Account #:	Ling, Susannah / 94556		
Account Number:	--		
Last Name:	Ling	Address 1:	234 Capeside Dr
First Name:	Susannah	Address 2:	--
Middle Initial:	--	City:	Anytown
Date of Birth:	01/02/1973	State:	AL
Age:	43	Zip:	12345
Sex:	Female	Email:	susannah.ling@scmo.edu
SSN:	111-22-3333	Home Phone:	445-555-7897
Employer Name:	Seaside Florist	Cell Phone:	--------

PROVIDER INFORMATION

Primary Provider:	James A. Martin, MD	Provider's Address 1:	1234 Anystreet
Referring Provider:	--	Provider's Address 2:	--
Date of Last Visit:	01/25/2014	City:	Anytown
Phone:	123-123-1234	State:	AL
		Zip:	12345

INSURANCE INFORMATION (If the patient is not the Insured party, please include date of birth for claims.)

Insurance:	Aetna	Claims Address 1:	1234 Insurance Way
Name of Policy Holder:	Susannah Ling	City:	Anytown
SSN:	111-22-3333	State:	AL
Policy/ID Number:	YYT5782251	Zip:	12345
Group Number:	AT12005	Claims Phone:	800-123-2222

PATIENT INFORMATION (Please use full legal name.)

Last Name:	Murray JR	Address 1:	115 Cartwright Dr
First Name:	Chase	Address 2:	--
Middle Initial:	B	City:	Anytown
Medical Record Number:	--	State:	AL
Date of Birth:	04/07/1993	Zip:	12345
Age:	21	Email:	chaser@zoom.edu
Sex:	Male	Home Phone:	970-840-1199
SSN:	630-58-4125	Driver's License:	87954285
Emergency Contact Name:	Roberta Murray	Emergency Contact Phone:	970-840-1199
Mother's Date of Birth:	04/18/1967	Mother's SSN:	654-78-9321
Mother's Work Phone:	852-788-9852		

GUARANTOR INFORMATION (Please use full legal name.)

Relationship of Guarantor to Patient:	Parent	Guarantor/Account #:	Murray, Roberta / 76320
		Account Number:	76320
Last Name:	Murray	Address 1:	115 Cartwright Dr
First Name:	Roberta	Address 2:	--
Middle Initial:	--	City:	Anytown
Date of Birth:	04/18/1967	State:	AL
Age:	46	Zip:	89754
Sex:	Female	Email:	--
SSN:	654-78-3210	Home Phone:	852-788-9852
Employer Name:	Hammer Heads Eatery	Cell Phone:	970-788-2250

PROVIDER INFORMATION

Primary Provider:	Julie Walden, MD	Provider's Address 1:	1234 Anystreet
Referring Provider:	--	Provider's Address 2:	--
Date of Last Visit:	08/2009	City:	Anytown
Phone:	123-123-1234	State:	AL
		Zip:	12345

INSURANCE INFORMATION (If the patient is not the Insured party, please include date of birth for claims.)

Insurance:	Aetna	Claims Address 1:	1234 Insurance Way
Name of Policy Holder:	Roberta Murray	City:	Anytown
SSN:	654-78-9321	State:	AL
Policy/ID Number:	77700142	Zip:	12345
Group Number:	UR4534	Claims Phone:	800-123-2222

PATIENT INFORMATION (Please use full legal name.)

Last Name:	Green	Address 1:	800 Liberty Court
First Name:	Miles	Address 2:	--
Middle Initial:	R	City:	Seacrest
Medical Record Number:	--	State:	AK
Date of Birth:	01/01/1957	Zip:	54600
Age:	57	Email:	--
Sex:	Male	Home Phone:	831-555-1954
SSN:	456-58-7782	Driver's License:	--
Emergency Contact Name:	Luke Hand	Emergency Contact Phone:	314-555-1200

GUARANTOR INFORMATION (Please use full legal name.)

Relationship of Guarantor to Patient:	Self		
Guarantor/Account #:	Green, Miles R		
Account Number:	--		
Last Name:	Green	Address 1:	800 Liberty Court
First Name:	Miles	Address 2:	--
Middle Initial:	R	City:	Seacrest
Date of Birth:	01/01/1957	State:	AK
Age:	57	Zip:	54600
Sex:	Male	Email:	--
SSN:	456-58-7782	Home Phone:	831-555-1954
Employer Name:	Baker Corrections	Cell Phone:	--------

PROVIDER INFORMATION

Primary Provider:	Julie Walden, MD	Provider's Address 1:	1234 Anystreet
Referring Provider:	Carrie Peach, MD	Provider's Address 2:	--
Date of Last Visit:	2010	City:	Anytown
Phone:	123-123-1234	State:	AL
		Zip:	12345

INSURANCE INFORMATION (If the patient is not the Insured party, please include date of birth for claims.)

Insurance:	Blue Cross Blue Shield	Claims Address 1:	1234 Insurance Place
Name of Policy Holder:	Miles Green	Claims Address 1:	--
SSN:	456-58-7782	City:	Anytown
Policy/ID Number:	PT1234098	State:	AL
Group Number:	HC345	Zip:	12345
		Claims Phone:	800-123-1111

Glossary for Computer Novices

Term	Definition

General Hardware and Computing Terms

Term	Definition
Developer	A company that designs software with specific features and functionality and writes programming code to create the application
Keyboarding	In a word, typing. You don't have to zoom across the keyboard so fast you leave a wake, but it's helpful to type with more than just your index fingers.
Keyboard shortcut	Most tasks within an application, such as copying and pasting, can be accomplished either with a series of mouse clicks or with an alternative series of keystrokes. These keystroke combinations often use the Ctrl or Alt key plus a letter. Some examples include Ctrl+C to copy data, Ctrl+V to paste data, and Ctrl+X to cut data; the F1 key is the Help key.
Workstation	In its broadest sense, a workstation is anyplace within the medical practice, including remotely connected locations, that is equipped with a PC, laptop computer, tablet computer, or other networked device. Workstations are usually furnished and stocked with office supplies. They may be located in offices, in clinical areas, or at reception desks. Even a personal digital assistant (PDA), such as an iPhone, can be considered a workstation.

General Software Terms

Term	Definition
File	A unit of organization for data stored on a computer and containing program files, text, graphics, or some combination of these. For example, in SCMO, each patient's chart is composed of records from many different files. The patient's visit information is stored in one file, the patient's appointments in another, the patient's history and examination data in another, the patient's orders in another, the patient's diagnoses in another, the patient's instructions in another, etc. A folder is a larger unit of organization than a file; files are kept in folders.
Icon	Like a blue highway sign with a white H indicating a nearby hospital, icons are miniature visual representations of tasks, commands, applications, functions, and other digital miscellany. They are part of programs we call *graphic user interfaces (GUIs)*. Clicking on an icon is generally more efficient than executing a keyboard command (but not always—see *Keyboard shortcut*).

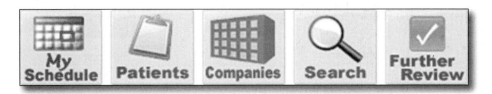

Term	Definition
Toolbar	A collection of icons (see *Icon*) arranged in a row and used as a graphic navigational aid. Toolbars are often *context specific*. This means that the toolbar you see shows only the icons appropriate for the screen on which you're working.

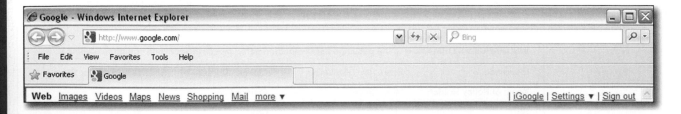

Term	Definition
Windows	In the broad sense, a window is a framed viewing area or portion of a screen that separates one part of an application from another, such as one file from another. A window can also separate one application from another. Using buttons in the upper right corner, each window can be closed (by clicking the black X), minimized—that is, made smaller (by clicking the single white line on the blue ground), or maximized—that is, resized to fill the entire computer display screen (by clicking the overlapping document icon or the large document icon). Navigational arrows (see *Back button and Forward arrow*) allow the user to move freely from window to window, minimizing and maximizing at will. Clicking the white X on the red background closes the entire program rather than just the current document. Windows can also be split, tiled, viewed side by side, and manipulated in other ways.

Glossary for Computer Novices—cont'd

Term	Definition
General Web/Internet Terms	
Browser (also called Internet browser or web browser)	An application that allows you to view and download content from the Internet (the web). The four most popular browsers are Firefox, Internet Explorer, Chrome, and Safari.
Home page	The main page (usually the opening screen) of a website. It contains general information and navigational links, such as a search box, sidebar menus, and links to subpages. In the earlier days of the Internet, home pages used to be more like book covers, offering little information beyond the name of the site. But these "landing pages" or "splash pages" just made it harder for visitors to access the content, and few sites have them anymore. An exception is a paid advertisement that may pop up over the home page (click Close or Skip This Ad to delete it). See *Website/web page*.

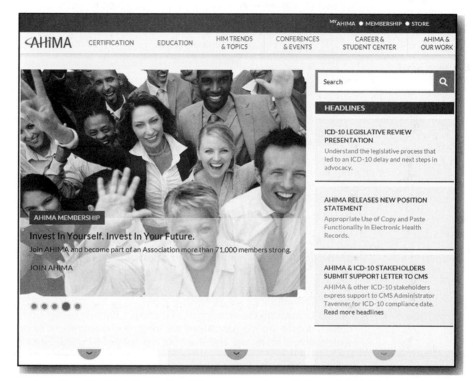

American Health Information Management Association's (AHIMA) home page.

Continued

Glossary for Computer Novices—cont'd

Term	Definition
Hyperlink (also called a link, live link, or hotlink)	An underlined web address, word, or phrase coded to jump to a new document, such as a website, or to a different part of the current document, or to select a function within SCMO. The link is activated when you click on it with your mouse (sometimes you must also press Ctrl while clicking).

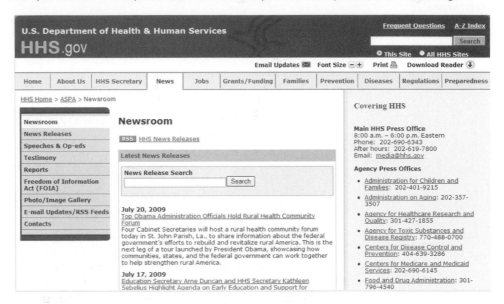

Each of the words and phrases underlined is a hyperlink. Clicking on any of the links takes you to the document described.

Term	Definition
Popup window	This term usually refers to the annoying ads that pop up on many commercial (.com) websites. However, within a software application such as an EHR, a popup screen or popup window is the same as a dialog box (see *Dialog box*).
URL	Uniform resource locator, or website address.
Website/web page	A specific location on the web, organized under a domain name. Commercial sites are .coms (dotcoms), not-for-profit organizations are .orgs, and government sites are .govs. Other domain-name extensions, such as .us, also exist but are not widely used. See *Home page.*

Glossary for Computer Novices—cont'd

Term	Definition
Document and Site Navigation and Manipulation Terms	
Back button and Forward arrow	Navigational icons, usually located in the upper left corner of a web browser or other application, used to move to the next page or screen of a document (Forward arrow) or to the previous page or screen (Back button).
Drag and drop	A function that allows you to shuffle text in a sentence or to reposition whole sentences. Just highlight the text you'd like to move (see *Highlight*), hold the mouse pointer over it, and drag it to the desired new position. To copy the text rather than move it, hold the Ctrl key as you drag. This function works for images as well.
Drop-down menu	A menu of further choices that appears (drops down) when a word on the menu bar is clicked. Many SCMO functions have a drop-down menu. In the Clinical Care module, Allergies, Medications, and Order Entry records are just a few examples of where drop-down menus are used.
Minimize/maximize/resize	To decrease *(minimize)* or increase *(maximize)* a window so that it fills only a portion of the computer monitor screen or the entire screen, respectively. To *resize* means to manipulate the size of a window or its position on the screen by minimizing or maximizing it or by using the "grab bars" on a graphic to expand or reduce its size. See *Windows*.
Undo/redo	These buttons, found in most applications, are quick editing tools that allow you to reverse a step or series of steps (by clicking Undo) and to perform them again, if you wish, by clicking Redo.
Scroll bar	Clickable up and down arrows or left and right arrows on a vertical bar. They are the graphic equivalent of the up, down, left, and right arrows on the keyboard. Scroll bars indicate that more text is available than would fit on the screen. They're used to navigate through documents and to browse through lists.
Data Input Terms	
Check box	A data input choice used when there are only two possible answers. A checked box generally means "yes" or "applicable," whereas an unchecked (blank) box means "no" or "not applicable." For example, a checkmarked box next to Cancel means "yes." To check or uncheck a box, click it once with the mouse.
Copy and paste	An editing function that allows you to highlight text or graphics and make an exact copy to be used elsewhere in your document or in another document.
Cut and paste	An editing function that allows you to highlight text or graphics and move the selected item elsewhere in your document or to another document.
Dialog box	A popup box that does one of three things: (1) contains additional information (called an alert box); (2) asks you to confirm that you wish to proceed (called a confirmation box); or (3) prompts you for more information (called a prompt box). See *Popup window*.
Highlight	Select a word, sentence, or passage to be edited (for example, moved, reformatted, or deleted) by clicking the right mouse button, dragging it across and down, and then releasing the button. Highlighted text is normally shown as white characters on a black background.

chapter 3

Privacy, Confidentiality, and Security

Chapter Outline

Commission on Accreditation of Allied Health Education Programs (CAAHEP) Competencies

1. Explore the issue of confidentiality as it applies to the medical assistant.
2. Describe the implications of HIPAA for the medical assistant in various medical settings.
3. Respond to issues of confidentiality.
4. Apply Health Insurance Portability and Accountability Act (HIPAA) of 1996 rules in regard to privacy/release of information.
5. Summarize the patient's bill of rights.
6. Recognize the importance of local, state, and federal legislation and regulations in the practice setting.

Chapter Objectives

1. Discuss privacy as both a philosophic and legal concept.
2. Explore the history and scope of HIPAA.

3. List the four implementation specifications required by the administrative safeguards outlined in the HIPAA Security Rule, and explore ways in which they might apply to a small to medium-size medical practice.

4. Assess and complete forms related to patient privacy and security in the electronic health record (EHR).

5. Become familiar with patients' rights under HIPAA, and explore how they affect the EHR.

6. Identify organizations aimed at securing EHR systems.

7. Identify who is allowed access to the information in a patient's EHR and under what circumstances.

8. Describe the role of consumer reporting agencies and prescription database tools, and explain how they are regulated.

9. Discuss ways patients can protect their health information.

Key Terms

adverse action   A decision by an insurance company, such as a health or disability insurer, to deny or terminate insurance or to increase rates, usually based on information obtained from a consumer reporting agency.

anonymity   The patient's right, which exists to varying degrees, to have private health data collected in a way that can never be linked or traced back to him or her.

audit trail   A record that traces a user's electronic footsteps by recording activity and transactions, including unsuccessful attempts to view unauthorized screens, within the EHR system.

authentication   The process of determining whether the person attempting to access a given network or EHR system is authorized to do so. User authentication can include password entry or use of biometric data (such as a digital fingerprint or voice signature) or a smart card (a data-laden microchip).

authorization   A document giving a covered entity permission to use protected health information for specified purposes other than treatment, payment, or healthcare operations or to disclose protected health information to a third party specified by the patient.

confidentiality   The patient's right and expectation that individually identifiable health information will be kept private and not disclosed without the patient's permission. Confidentiality is limited or protected by law to varying degrees.

consent   Permission given to a covered entity for uses and disclosures of protected health information for treatment, payment, and healthcare operations.

consumer reporting agency   An agency regulated by the Federal Trade Commission (FTC) under the Fair Credit Reporting Act (FCRA) that sells or cooperatively exchanges consumer information and history in areas such as credit and healthcare.

covered entities   Healthcare providers, health plans, and healthcare clearinghouses that transmit claims electronically. As part of covered entities, business associates are those who are contracted by covered entities to perform specific duties and have a corresponding contract detailing their responsibilities.

disclosure   Giving access to, releasing, or transferring information to a person or entity not legally or ethically authorized to use or have knowledge of it.

ethics   Rules and standards of conduct that govern professional behavior and arise from our shared understanding of morality.

individually identifiable health information (IIHI)   Health information that clearly identifies an individual patient or could reasonably be used to identify the patient; see *protected health information (PHI)*.

laws   Formal, enforceable rules and policies based on community standards of conduct.

minimum necessary standard   A key provision of the HIPAA Privacy Rule requiring that disclosures include no more than the minimum necessary amount of information to accomplish a given purpose.

off-label indication   A use for a prescription drug other than that for which the U.S. Food and Drug Administration (FDA) has approved it.

password A sequence of characters and sometimes spaces used to prevent unauthorized access to or disclosure of patient information contained in secure electronic files.

privacy The patient's freedom to determine when, how much, and under what circumstances his or her medical information may be disclosed.

protected health information (PHI) Individually identifiable health information that is stored, maintained, or transmitted electronically; in practice, however, this term is often used interchangeably with the term IIHI, regardless of what form the information takes.

safeguards Measures taken to prevent interference with computer network operations and to avert security breaches involving the unauthorized use, disclosure, modification, erasure, or destruction of protected health information; these measures are specified by the HIPAA Security Rule, which applies only to data in electronic form.

screensaver A program that displays moving text or images on the screen if input (such as a keystroke) is not received for a given time period.

secondary use A use of health information that is not directly related to patient care. Such uses include statistical analysis, research, quality and safety assurance processes, public health monitoring, payment, provider certification or accreditation, and marketing and other business activities.

WHAT IS PRIVACY?

New technology in the medical office, including the EHR, has changed the way patients' **privacy,** confidentiality, and security are maintained. We all have a general idea of what these concepts mean—who doesn't know what privacy is? But concepts and principles that often seem abstract actually have specific meaning within the legal system. They are put in place to protect consumers and patients from those who might want to use their information for harm. Now that everything from bank card numbers to patient test results are stored online, maintaining privacy has become even more difficult.

Both law and ethics, sometimes a little more of one than the other, require that patients be treated with respect and dignity and be offered the best care we're capable of providing given the time and budgetary constraints that always exist. **Ethics** is the set of rules and standards of conduct that grow out of our shared understanding of right and wrong and that govern our professional behavior. When we formalize (codify) these ethical principles and determine criminal or civil penalties for violating them, we call them **laws.**

Before we define a few more concepts, let's make sure we keep our discussion concrete by seeing how they might apply to real patients. Edmund is a 64-year-old writer of fiction and biography who has made something of a name for himself. Ed has been openly gay for many years and knows he is human immunodeficiency virus (HIV) positive. Ed's partner, a 51-year-old electrical engineer named Michael, has chosen to share his sexual orientation with the couple's wide circle of friends but not with his elderly parents. Michael would like to be tested periodically for HIV, but he is concerned about his privacy. In other words, Michael would like to decide when, how much, and with whom his medical information can be shared.

CRITICAL THINKING EXERCISE 3-1

Do you agree with the idea that it's human nature to show a preference, at times, for those we like or have something in common with and to be occasionally less attentive to those we find disagreeable or who are least like us? If so, what can we do as ethical healthcare professionals to treat patients equitably? Or do you think it's all right to show a preference?

Confidential Versus Anonymous

Although the terms are often used interchangeably, a confidential test like the HIV test Michael has requested is not the same thing as an anonymous test. To adequately protect patients' privacy, it's important to know the difference. **Confidentiality** refers to how the recipient of the information, such as Michael's physician, handles information that a patient does not wish to have disclosed.

The notion of confidentiality presumes that the person is entitled to keep the information to himself or herself and that the provider or other person with whom the information is shared is obligated to hold it in confidence. This is often not the case. For instance, suspected child abuse must be reported to law enforcement. Sexual assault and other crimes may also be subject to reporting requirements. In some states, minors who seek family planning advice or services may be reported to parents or guardians. HIV and certain other communicable diseases, as in Michael's case, are subject to state reporting requirements so that partners can be notified and disease incidence can be tracked for public health purposes.

Confidential information may be disclosed to other parties besides public health and law enforcement officials. If Michael agrees to disclose his test results to his physician, who would then enter the information into the EHR, his test results would undoubtedly reach Michael's health insurance company. Why? Because to obtain health insurance, even for a group plan, he would have had to sign a document permitting them access to his health records.

If Michael prefers to have an anonymous test, he may be able to get one at a local public health clinic. **Anonymity** means that Michael's name will not be linked to the results. His blood sample will be submitted to the lab using only an identification number, and a counselor will share the results with him by phone.

HEALTH INSURANCE PORTABILITY AND ACCOUNTABILITY ACT (HIPAA)

The electronic age has made our lives easier, safer, and more rewarding in many ways. Yet technology also poses problems that were inconceivable just a generation or two ago. Publishers used to worry about illegal distribution of photocopies; now they must patrol the Internet to make sure their copyrighted material hasn't become accessible to millions of people worldwide. Drug enforcement officials who used to police street corners are now charged with keeping prescription narcotics from being sold online and delivered right to the purchaser's door. And in many cities, the number of fender-benders has spiked as drivers, fearful that they'll be captured by a red-light camera if they proceed through the intersection, slam on their brakes the moment the light turns yellow.

Citizens and elected officials have struggled to sort out issues like these in every area of our lives, including healthcare and privacy. In times past, only a small number of medical personnel had access to patients' paper charts, but when electronic transmission of data became possible, health information quickly became an easily exchanged commodity. Some insurers began to deny patients coverage because of preexisting conditions, which could be quickly verified via electronic means. In response, Congress passed the Health Insurance Portability and Accountability Act of 1996, which prohibited such denials as long as a person could prove prior continuous health insurance coverage. The scope of the law has since been expanded. As we know it today, HIPAA not only makes health insurance portable but also protects privacy and security.

To standardize the process of data submission and collection as people moved and changed names, an amendment to HIPAA established a set of codes for claims transmitted electronically. Each provider, employer, and health plan was assigned its own identification number. The idea of having patients' health information linked to their Social Security number imposed a high level of vulnerability to privacy intrusions and security threats. The HIPAA Privacy Rule was passed to shore up this weakness.

TRENDS AND APPLICATIONS 3-1

Can Patients' Genetic Profiles Be Used Against Them?

One public concern that has delayed the transition to a nationwide system of EHR systems is the fear of genetic discrimination. This kind of discrimination occurs when an employer, insurer, or other party discriminates against a patient or family member based on the genetic predisposition to develop a given illness. For example, an insurer might wish to drop coverage for a family that receives a preterm diagnosis of cystic fibrosis. Certain types of genetic discrimination are merely theoretic. Some patients and privacy advocates worry that testing could be used to discriminate against people in employment and other matters. Tens of thousands of genetic paternity tests have already been done without consent, points out the ACLU, and it's impossible to tell what other kinds of "genetic spying," medical or otherwise, might be possible in the future. J. Lo's genome on Facebook, perhaps?

Privacy concerns about patients' genetic information are pitting patients and physicians against insurers and employers. Patients want to keep genetic information private, but insurers don't want to shoulder the burden of policyholders who are likely to become ill, and employers want to hire healthy employees whose health insurance premiums are low.

Testing is available for about 1500 genetic disorders, and that figure is continually increasing. Amniocentesis procedures generally screen for Down syndrome, Tay-Sachs disease, sickle cell disease, cystic fibrosis, neural tube defects, thalassemia, or some combination of those diseases, depending on the parents' risk factors. Although it may not be necessary, practical, or cost effective to do so, genes for any of these diseases can be detected while a fetus is still in the womb or even before an embryo fertilized in a lab is transferred to a woman's uterus. However, many genetic tests cannot determine whether a person will definitely develop a given disease—only whether the person is likely to do so. Those who carry a gene for schizophrenia, for example, have a 50/50 chance of developing the disease, with environmental factors making up the other half of the equation.

Genetic testing has the potential to help patients and providers make sound treatment decisions, aid researchers who are looking for new links between genetic mutations and disease development, lower costs for insurance companies by preventing disease (for example, in patients who undergo preventive mastectomies), and increase worker productivity for employers by reducing days off and leaves of absence for illness. Despite these obvious benefits, however, a 2004 study of patients with a family history of colorectal cancer showed that many of them would not only refuse genetic testing but said they would not even agree to speak with a healthcare professional about their family history for fear the information would be used against them in employment and insurance coverage decisions.

According to a survey conducted by the Johns Hopkins Genetics and Public Policy Center, 93% of Americans believe that neither their insurance companies nor their employers should have access to the results of genetic tests. Yet the American public does agree that gathering genetic information is important. The same survey found that almost as many respondents—91%—said that if effective treatment were available for a particular condition, they would entrust their physicians (but not necessarily anyone else) with the genetic information necessary to diagnose and treat it.

Furthermore, new parents believe it's important to collect genetic health information about their newborns. A 2007 poll conducted by the C. S. Mott Children's Hospital at the University of Michigan found that 54% of parents approve of genetic testing even for diseases for which no effective treatment is available. In addition, 38% of parents said they would allow their child's genetic information to be linked to a nationally interoperable EHR system. Such a system would undoubtedly be an invaluable public health resource, but it would have to address the valid privacy concerns we've just discussed.

In an effort to begin addressing such concerns, in 2008, Congress passed the Genetic Information Nondiscrimination Act (GINA). Individuals who have group health insurance were already protected, but GINA extends protection to those who own individual insurance policies. Health insurers will be prohibited from raising premiums or denying coverage based on a person's genetic risk profile, and employers may not fire an employee or discriminate in hiring, promotion, or compensation on that basis.

Privacy Rule

The HIPAA Privacy Rule establishes privacy standards for the use and disclosure of **individually identifiable health information (IIHI)**, promotes patients' understanding of their privacy rights, and helps patients control the ways in which their health information is used and disclosed. The rule aims to balance the necessity of making important health disclosures to authorized persons or entities against the patient's right to privacy in the healthcare arena.

Unlike other provisions of HIPAA, the HIPAA Privacy Rule applies to health information in any form—in conversation, on paper, or in electronic format. **Protected health information (PHI),** on the other hand, refers to any IIHI stored, maintained, or transmitted electronically. In practice, however, these terms are often used interchangeably.

The Privacy Rule, which took effect in 2003, specifies that each time PHI is released for a purpose other than treatment, payment, or other healthcare operations, the **disclosure** must be documented and a record of it maintained for 6 years. Patients are permitted to request a log of such disclosures, which must include the following for each disclosure:

- The date of the disclosure
- The name and address, if known, of the entity or person who received the IIHI
- A description of the IIHI disclosed
- An explanation of the purpose of the disclosure or a copy of the patient's written authorization
- A copy of a written request for a disclosure, if any

The rule also requires any provider or other entity subject to the rule to do the following:

- Distribute notices informing patients of the provider's privacy practices, including its policies for handling information contained in the patient's EHR
- Designate a privacy official to oversee adoption of privacy policies and procedures and to ensure compliance with them. In a small office this might be a staff member with other duties as well, such as an office manager. Figure 3-1 is a detailed job description of a privacy official in a medical office.
- Offer authorization forms for release of PHI
- Implement policies to protect patients' records and to give patients access to their records
- Develop procedures for amending records when they are found to be in error
- Certify that staff members or employees have been trained in HIPAA Privacy Rule standards and in the provider's privacy practices. In a small office, training may consist of simply handing out the office privacy policy and documenting that all staff members have reviewed it and understand it. Larger practices might provide instruction or ask staff members to complete a self-paced online HIPAA course.

EHR EXERCISE 3-1:   DISCLOSURE AUTHORIZATION

*Complete the following exercise in the EHR Exercises environment of SimChart for the Medical Office.

Erma Willis (12/09/1947) is a patient of Dr. Martin and has been asked to participate in a stroke prevention study conducted by the Heart Wellness and Research Group at 345 Vascula Lane, Anytown, AL 12345. In order to participate, Ms. Willis must provide copies of any lipid panels and ECGs from the past 10 years. Use SCMO to prepare a Disclosure Authorization for Ms. Willis. The signature on file is dated as today and this authorization will expire 1 year from today's date.

1. Select the Disclosure Authorization from the left info panel of the Form Repository and use the Patient Search button to link the document to the patient record before proceeding.

2. Fill in the blank text fields and save the completed document to the patient record using the Save to Patient Record button.

Figure 3-1
A sample job description of a privacy official in a medical office.

JOB DESCRIPTION
HIPAA SECURITY OFFICER
Complete Health Care Associates

Reports to: The security officer reports to Complete Health Care Associates.

Summary: The HIPAA security officer is responsible for overseeing the development and implementation of Complete Health Care Associate's security policies and practices. The security officer is responsible for coordinating all of the practice's activities that have security implications. In addition, the security officer is responsible for monitoring the practice's services and systems to ensure it has meaningful practices with regard to security. The security officer is also responsible for advocating and protecting the security of electronic protected health information related to the practice's patients.

Essential duties and responsibilities

• Reports to Complete Health Care Associates on current and emerging federal and state legislation and regulations impacting security. Makes recommendations as to how the practice should comply with these regulations.

• Keeps Complete Health Care Associates apprised as to the status of the practice's implementation of security procedures.

• Documents the practice's security procedures.

• Monitors compliance with the practice's security policies. Responsible for documenting and responding to any problems that occur.

• Conducts security risk assessments and audits for the practice.

• Monitors internal controls to ensure that information access levels and security clearances are maintained.

• Prepares the practice's disaster recovery and emergency mode operation plans for information systems.

• Develops an employee training program regarding security requirements. Ensures that all new employees are trained within 30 days of their employment with the practice.

• Ensures that the practice appropriately protects and maintains patient information.

• Keeps abreast of new developments regarding HIPAA security and monitors any changes in the regulations.

• Maintains employees' security awareness through reminders and updates.

Qualifications

Must have strong technical skills (operating systems, hardware, security measures, firewalls, etc.).

Must have detailed knowledge of the practice's information systems and flow of electronic protected health information.

Must have good communication skills and leadership ability.

Must possess high level of integrity and trust.

Must possess excellent follow-up and documentation skills.

Must have conflict resolution skills.

Must possess ability to assess business risks and enforce appropriate security measures.

Must possess in-depth knowledge of the HIPAA Security Rule.

CRITICAL THINKING EXERCISE 3-2

Mr. Rogers, a letter carrier for the U.S. Postal Service, has developed a serious bloodstream infection after a Yorkshire terrier bit him on the ankle. Mr. Rogers's physician and nurse are discussing the patient's condition and history at his bedside. Mr. Edelman, the patient in the next bed, overhears the entire conversation, including the somewhat embarrassing story of how Mr. Rogers lost a fingertip 8 years ago after offering a leftover chicken nugget to a cocker spaniel on his route. Have the physician and nurse violated the HIPAA Privacy Rule?

Covered Entities and Business Associates

Only **covered entities**—healthcare providers, health plans, and healthcare clearinghouses—are subject to the HIPAA Privacy Rule:

- Under the rule, the term *healthcare provider* refers broadly to any business within the healthcare industry that transmits claims electronically. Thus even medical laboratories and accounting firms that process medical bills are considered to be providers. Although it's theoretically possible for a medical practice to circumvent HIPAA by submitting claims only on paper, it would be difficult to do so because even the practice's subcontractors, such as billing agencies, would also have to submit paper claims. If the providers within the practice had any hospital affiliations, electronic transmission would be a near certainty.

- The term *health plan* is subject to a similarly open interpretation under the rule. Almost any payer of medical costs, such as Medicare or a union-sponsored health insurance plan, is considered to be a health plan. Notable exceptions, however, include law enforcement agencies (in certain circumstances), workers' compensation, and vehicle insurance policies that offer injury coverage.

- A *healthcare clearinghouse* is an information-processing company that allows healthcare services and billing companies with incompatible platforms to share data.

The HIPAA Privacy Rule also applies to business associates. Business associates are entities who help to carry out the healthcare activities and operations of the medical office. The business associate may be a subcontractor who creates, receives, maintains, or transmits protected health information on behalf of the covered entity. The covered entity is responsible for establishing a written contract with the business associate that outlines the specific requirements and responsibilities. The contract outlines the privacy and security requirements of protected health information.

Minimum Necessary

The HIPAA Privacy Rule centers on a privacy standard known as the **minimum necessary standard.** According to this provision, when a covered entity makes an allowed disclosure, it should include only the minimum necessary amount of information to accomplish the purpose at hand. The standard does not apply to disclosures made to the patient, disclosures made to other healthcare providers, disclosures the patient has authorized (see the following section), or disclosures made in certain other circumstances. For example, the rule allows—but doesn't require—an exception to be made for requesting parties on which the covered entity may have so-called reasonable reliance, such as a public official who needs the information for public health purposes, another covered entity, or a legitimate researcher.

The Privacy Rule requires healthcare personnel to take reasonable precautions not to discuss patients' personal information where it might be overheard, such as in elevators and reception areas, at cashiers' windows, and so on. However, the rule does not prohibit discussion of patient information in treatment areas, at pharmacy counters, and over the phone as long as reasonable precautions, such as lowering your voice, are taken.

Consent Versus Authorization

The HIPAA Privacy Rule rests on the so-called *individual choice principle,* which states that patients should have a reasonable opportunity to make informed decisions about the collection, use, and disclosure of their IIHI. For example, Michael would like his physician to be able to discuss his test results with Ed but not with his parents. To accomplish this, Michael signs an **authorization** form, which—somewhat contrary to common sense—can be used to revoke as well as to grant permission to disclose IIHI. An authorization form is needed when information is to be disclosed for purposes other than treatment, payment, or operations (such as for training or for quality assurance analysis). A general authorization is usually adequate, but a specific authorization is required to disclose information considered especially sensitive, such as the results of an HIV test. An authorization form includes the components listed in Box 3-1. No authorization is required for certain kinds of disclosures, and other disclosures may be made by the patient voluntarily.

BOX 3-1
Components of an Authorization Form

- Complete name, date of birth, and address of the patient
- A description of the information to be disclosed (including specific dates) and for what purpose
- A description of the information that may not be disclosed
- The name of the individuals providing the information
- A list of individuals or entities to whom the information may be disclosed
- A date on which the disclosure expires
- A statement informing the patient that the authorization may be revoked if he or she changes his or her mind
- A notice advising the patient that the information disclosed could be redisclosed and therefore would no longer be protected
- The patient's signature and date signed

EHR EXERCISE 3-2: AUTHORIZATION FOR THE RELEASE OF MEDICAL RECORDS

*Complete the following exercise in the EHR Exercises environment of SimChart for the Medical Office.

Walter Biller (01/04/1970) is an established patient of Dr. Walden. He is scheduled to see an orthopedic specialist, Dr. Marian Brown, next Wednesday for treatment of left shoulder pain. Prior to that visit, Dr. Brown would like to review all medical records from 2013 to the present. The medical records release will expire in 90 days or immediately after it is complete. Dr. Marian Brown's office is located at Medical Arts Building, Suite 3B, Anytown, AL 12345. Dr. Brown's office phone is 123-878-8989 and fax is 123-690-2164. Prepare a Medical Records Release for the patient's signature.

1. Select the Medical Records Release from the left info panel of the Form Repository and use the Patient Search button to link the document to the patient record before proceeding.

2. Fill in the blank text fields and save the completed document to the patient record using the Save to Patient Record button.

Security Rule

Given the widespread use of electronic information-sharing technologies such as EHRs and computerized provider order entry (CPOE), as well as the goal of making such technologies nationally interoperable, public authorities saw a need to strengthen the security of PHI. The HIPAA Security Rule gives each covered entity four broad goals to meet:

1. Protect the integrity and confidentiality of electronic healthcare information created, received, maintained, or transmitted
2. Shield such information against security threats that can reasonably be anticipated
3. Shelter PHI against unauthorized use and disclosure, as outlined in the HIPAA Privacy Rule
4. Ensure that all employees comply with the provisions of the Security Rule

Privacy Versus Security

In plain English, the Security Rule is supposed to ensure that information is not destroyed by natural disaster or some more malicious means, and that only people who are supposed to have access to PHI can gain access to it that's in line with their job functions. As you can see from the third goal, the HIPAA Privacy and Security Rules are closely bound up with each other. So what's the difference? The HIPAA Privacy Rule governs the use and disclosure of PHI in all forms, whereas the HIPAA Security Rule outlines the administrative, physical, and technologic measures that covered entities must take in order to implement and comply with the Privacy Rule. In a nutshell, the Privacy Rule is a statement of principles and the Security Rule is a plan for applying them.

SECURITY SAFEGUARDS IN THE MEDICAL PRACTICE

The HIPAA Security Rule, which applies only to the patient's *electronic* health information, offers **safeguards** designed to avert security breaches and provide contingency plans in case network operations are interrupted. Safeguards fall into three areas: administrative, physical, and technical. Instead of laying out a rigid prescription for implementation, however, the Security Rule invites a range of approaches for complying with the standards. This flexibility allows each healthcare institution, provider, or health plan to carry out the provisions of the rule in a way that makes sense given its size, organizational complexity, technologic capabilities, budget, and the kinds of risks to which it's exposed. Let's see how the EHR figures into each kind of safeguard.

Administrative

Administrative safeguards require the medical practice or other covered entity to adopt formal processes to prevent, detect, contain, and correct security violations. These provisions are part of the Health Information Technology for Economic and Clinical Health (HITECH) Act meaningful use reporting requirements. The security management process comprises four implementation specifications:

1. **Risk analysis.** The medical office must assess threats to the confidentiality, integrity, and availability of PHI.
2. **Risk management.** The practice should put security measures in place in order to minimize risks to a level that can be managed effectively. Doing so requires strong leadership and good communication.
3. **Sanction (penalties) policy.** The practice must determine before any infraction occurs what the penalties will be for staff members who fail to comply with security measures. Penalties should increase in proportion to the severity of the offense.
4. **Information system activity review.** The office should construct a procedure to review its compliance procedures periodically. For example, after reviewing audit trails and security incident reports, it can revise policies to shore up any weaknesses in its security plan.

To carry out these implementation specifications, the practice must assign a security officer. The security officer is responsible for supervising the development and implementation of security policies, education, practices, and procedures and for coordinating all of the practice's activities that have security implications. The security officer is also responsible for advocating and protecting the security of PHI related to the practice's patients.

The officer should have detailed knowledge of HIPAA requirements and EHR systems. Like the privacy officer, the security officer may be an existing employee with other job responsibilities. In a larger practice the scope of the officer's responsibilities might warrant making it a separate, full-time position.

Physical

Covered entities, including the medical practice, must ensure the physical security of the electronic data, buildings, and equipment they maintain by guarding them against unauthorized intrusion and by shielding them from natural disasters and environmental hazards. The possibility of a national security emergency must also be considered.

Protection against unauthorized intrusion first requires securing the facility in which the EHR system is housed—for our purposes, the medical practice. This might mean using locks, security guards, employee identification and visitor badges, or video monitoring. Network security requires password protection and contingency planning for scheduled downtime, system outages, and data loss.

In addition, equipment must be protected from unauthorized access, tampering, and theft. For any workstation at which PHI can be accessed—and that includes all mobile devices!—the practice must specify which security procedures limit access to patient databases. To do so, threats to desktop computers and laptops must be assessed. The practice must specify where each laptop or desktop computer may be placed or used and must incorporate security devices that limit unauthorized access, such as **screensavers.** A screensaver is a program that displays moving text or images on a screen if no input, such as a keystroke, is received for a given time period (typically a few minutes). Patient information should never be left unattended on a computer screen, where any passerby could view, change, or retrieve a patient's EHR. Screensavers limit unauthorized viewing of patient information while the user is away from his or her desk. When the user returns and strikes a key, the screensaver disappears and the EHR system can be accessed again. The staff must keep maintenance records indicating when screensavers and other such security devices are installed. In addition, systems will automatically log a user out of the system after a period of time with no activity.

The practice must design a plan for the receipt, removal, backup, storage, reuse, disposal, and accountability of electronic media, such as EHR systems stored on magnetic tape or disks and memory cards. Essentially the practice must know where its information has been, who it was with, and what it was doing there. Before any EHR is moved, an easily retrievable copy of it must be made.

Finally, the medical practice must have a plan to restore data in the event of a national emergency or natural disaster. Data must be backed up on a server (the practice's own or that of a vendor), and plans must be in place for alternative means of entering and accessing patients' records.

Login Procedures

Access to files can be limited using a secure, password-based login system such as that used in the SimChart for the Medical Office (SCMO). To help practices meet physical security specifications, only physicians and staff members with an appropriate **password** are able to access the program information. Passwords are character sequences chosen by the user and intended to prevent improper use or disclosure of patient information by preventing unauthorized access to records. However, a computer can verify only that the password is valid—it can't **authenticate** that the person using it is authorized to do so. Thus a strong password should be chosen (Box 3-2), should be kept in a secure place if written down at all, and should never be given to anyone else. Further steps may be required for user authentication, such as the entry of biometric data or the insertion of a smart card containing encoded user data.

> ### *BOX 3-2*
> **Tips for Choosing a Strong Password**
>
> The stronger your password, the less likely it is to be guessed by another person or detected by a computer program. Here are some tips:
> - Remember that the more characters you use, the stronger your password. Just think how much easier it would be to Pick 3 to win than to Pick 6 in the Lotto! A minimum of eight characters is recommended.
> - Choose a combination of letters, numbers, and symbols (asterisk, exclamation point, percentage sign, etc.).
> - Avoid using characters in sequence, such as ABC, 123, and 1111.
> - If your password is case sensitive (that is, the computer recognizes whether a letter is capitalized), choose both uppercase and lowercase characters.
> - If you have a Rottweiler named Warren, don't choose **warren1** as your password. If your new boyfriend's name is Carmine, don't use **carminerox** as your password. You get the picture—don't choose a password that can be easily guessed, including your name, Social Security number, wedding anniversary, birthday, or the birthdays of your children.
> - Don't choose words that are found in a dictionary. Instead, create "words" from the first letters of phrases you can remember. Thus "Warren is the best dog in the world!" becomes "**Witbditw!**" To make the password even more impenetrable, add numbers or swap a letter for a symbol.
> - Change your password often (and NEVER share it with anyone!).

Technical

The HIPAA Security Rule provides for technical safeguards that protect and control access to patients' PHI. In accordance with the Privacy Rule, the covered entity—again, for our purposes, the medical practice—must grant users the minimum necessary access to PHI they need to perform their job functions. Such a tiered system of access might give a nurse practitioner the ability to change the patient note and to refill prescriptions but deny the receptionist those same privileges.

A description of each employee's access to the EHR should be listed in the policies and procedures manual of the medical office. This information can also be given in general terms that state what kind of access each *type* of employee (medical assistant, nurse, physician, and so on) is permitted to have. The student access in SCMO is one that a physician would have. This enables the student to access all of the same functionality in the EHR that a physician can access, including the patient's demographics, history and examination, order entry, diagnosing, patient education instructions, and billing functions. However, EHR systems allow access to specific items to be limited. For example, certain blood test results, like in Michael's HIV case, may be viewed only by the treating physician.

To create this kind of system, users must have unique usernames or numbers, and procedures for emergency access must be in place. (This part of the technical specification overlaps with the physical specification, which addresses passwords and emergency contingency plans.) Optional security measures might include automatic logoff after a period of inactivity or encryption (scrambling data into code) and decryption (translating the coded data) technology. A procedure must also be designated to terminate access by those who are no longer authorized to use the information.

> ## CRITICAL THINKING EXERCISE 3-3
>
> Name several situations in which it would be dangerous to the patient if a key piece of his or her health information were changed or deleted, either intentionally or inadvertently.

Assigning Employee Privileges

Figure 3-2 shows an example of an access log for a physician's office. This log provides an explanation of employee access to the EHR. The log details the name of the employee, job title, description of physical access (full or limited), and start date of access. Once the staff member leaves the employ of the medical office, the date of termination is documented as well.

EMPLOYEE ACCESS LOG

Employee Name	Description of Access (systems, building, files, etc.)	Full or Limited Access (if limited, explain)	Login/ PW	Date of Access	Date Access Removed	Deleted Login PW (√)	Retrieved Keys, Cards, etc. (√)
Jane Andrew	Medical Records Technician: Building A&B, file rooms, EHR	Limited EHR access: unable to change notes or e-prescribing	Login: Ja_files PW: XX215	01/12/XX			
Jose Martinez	Nurse: Building A&B, EHR	Full Access	Login: Jm_nurse PW: REHCC	02/04/XX			

Figure 3-2 An example of an access log for a physician's office.

CRITICAL THINKING EXERCISE 3-4

You are the practice manager for a prominent Beverly Hills plastic surgeon, and you overhear your staff talking about the nose j—er, that is, the rhinoplasty—of a high-profile patient seen in your office. You hold an emergency staff meeting at the end of the day to approach those you suspect leaked the information. Everyone denies having been the source of the gossip. How can you prove your suspicions?

Designing Auditing Procedures

Technical safeguards also include **audit trails,** systems tied to a person's username or password that reveal the electronic breadcrumb trail each of us leaves behind as we move through the EHR system. This trail helps ensure the integrity—that is, the correctness and completeness—of the data. After all, patient records are not supposed to be like Wikipedia entries, in which anyone who has a mind to add, change, or delete a patient's health information can just go in and do so.

Periodically the security officer should examine each employee's access trail within the EHR. The audit or login function within SCMO allows the provider or practice manager (or in this case professor) to view all modifications to a patient's record. This is typically the role of an administrative officer and not a general job responsibility of the usual EHR user.

Limited-Access Policies for Specific Patients

Access to individual patient records can be designated as well, allowing only specified groups of staff members to view that patient's PHI. Let's say you work at a medical spa where Bobby Trendy gets Botox injections and an occasional chemical peel. Within the patient's chart, you can assign Trendy to one or more specific groups that would contain only those users who have the authority to view his chart. When this feature is set, Trendy will not show up in patient searches conducted by users outside the specified group(s). This is a customizable feature that can be set for every patient chart.

Limiting employee access to patient information is only one way of increasing patient privacy. Patients can also control who has access to their health information. The medical office staff will document *disclosure information, alternative means*. An alternative means document states the patients' preference for where they may be contacted and whether they allow anyone else to have access to their medical information (their spouse, for example). The medical staff can also document when a patient was given the notice of privacy practice (NPP) forms.

EHR EXERCISE 3-3: NOTICE OF PRIVACY PRACTICE (NPP) AND PATIENT'S BILL OF RIGHTS DOCUMENTS

*Complete the following exercise in the EHR Exercises environment of SimChart for the Medical Office.

Susannah Ling (01-02-1973) has come into the office today to drop off completed new patient paperwork before her first appointment next week. As the medical assistant, you will provide Susannah with a copy of the NPP and patient's bill of rights documents.

The office procedure is to save the documents to her patient record as acknowledgment. Use the Form Repository to link and print these documents to the patient record:

1. Click the Form Repository icon and select the NPP from the left info panel (Figure 3-3).

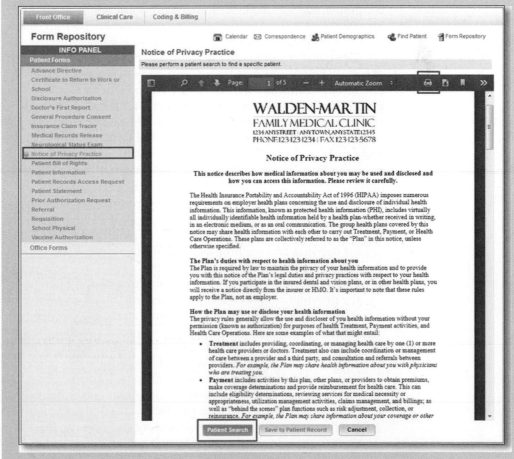

Figure 3-3   NPP form with the form location, Patient Search button, and Print icon called out.

> **2.** Click the Patient Search button at the bottom of the form to search for Susannah Ling's record.
>
> **3.** Once you select Susannah's record, you can use the Save to Record button to store the form in the patient's record. Use the Print icon to provide the patient a copy.
>
> **4.** Now select the Patient Bill of Rights from the Form Repository, directly below the NPP.
>
> You may access these forms at any time to view or print in the Patient Dashboard in the Clinical Care module.

PATIENTS' RIGHTS UNDER HIPAA

Even with the best of intentions, government regulations are usually tangled up in red tape, and HIPAA is no exception. The original law, passed in 1996, has been amended numerous times. In fact, the 2006 HIPAA Administrative Simplification document, also known as Title II, runs 101 pages. That's nearly four times as long as the HIPAA Privacy Rule, which took effect in 2003. As a result, HIPAA is often misinterpreted, not only by patients but also by healthcare personnel, resulting in misunderstanding. According to *The New York Times*, an Arizona nursing home put an end to birthday parties for residents because they believed revealing birth dates was a HIPAA violation. Physicians' unwarranted reluctance to release children's immunization records has stymied the creation of immunization registries nationwide. And one transplant surgeon was denied information about a donor heart because the donor's medical team did not want to violate the recently deceased patient's privacy.

It's easy to be intimidated by the law or, frankly, bored by the monotonous legalese of privacy notices, compliance data, authorization forms, and the like. Nevertheless, as caring members of the healthcare community, we must all understand how to enforce the provisions of HIPAA without going overboard. After all, it's a real law that affects real people who make up the patient populations we serve.

Ellen, a 37-year-old with multiple sclerosis (MS), is one of them. After suffering a series of complications during a recent flare-up of her disease, Ellen decided to take a more active role in her healthcare. One of her first steps was to request copies of her records from the physicians who have been treating her—a neurologist, ophthalmologist, gastroenterologist, and general practitioner (GP). All of the practices except Ellen's GP's office sent copies of her records promptly after receiving her written request. However, Tamara, the medical assistant at the GP's office, explained (in error, as Ellen soon learned) that HIPAA prohibits releasing Ellen's own records to her. As a result, Ellen investigated HIPAA regulations and quickly determined that she—and every other patient—has the right to the following:

- **View or receive copies of her health record.** Surprisingly, before the HIPAA Privacy Rule took effect, patients in some states could be denied access to their own health records. Now, although the insurer or medical practice may charge a reasonable fee for copying and mailing, as most of Ellen's physicians did, a patient's access to his or her own records is guaranteed by law.
- **Have inaccurate health information corrected.** If Ellen finds information that she and the provider agree is wrong, a correction (called an *amendment*) must be made within 60 days except under special circumstances. The erroneous information need not be removed from the file, but it must be made clear that the amended information supersedes it. And, of course, it must be obvious which is which. If the provider does not agree that the information is inaccurate, he or she is not required by HIPAA to remove or amend it. However, Ellen still has some recourse. She can file a *statement of disagreement* in her EHR to indicate which information she believes is inaccurate and why.
- **Receive a notice of privacy practices.** This notice explains how IIHI can be disclosed, to whom, and under what circumstances. Typically this notice is given to patients at their first visit with the physician. It is then documented either on the paper chart or in a note in the EHR.
- **Opt out of sharing certain information with certain people.** If you want your physician to be able to discuss your medical care with your mother but not your father or

with your wife but not your ex-wife, you can specify that preference, and your provider must honor any reasonable request. You can also choose, for example, to make your name and room number unavailable to the hospital switchboard or make any other privacy request that can reasonably be carried out.

- **Have certain information withheld from certain third parties.** In addition to the option to designate certain people from whom information should be withheld, as just described, HIPAA specifies that Ellen's health information will *automatically* be kept confidential from her employer, direct marketers, and others unless she signs an authorization form to release the information to them.
- **Receive a list of disclosures of her health information.** Ellen can find out who has accessed her EHR as well as when and why.
- **File a complaint.** If Ellen believes that any of her providers have violated the provisions of HIPAA, she has the right to file a complaint with the Office for Civil Rights (OCR) of the U.S. Department of Health and Human Services (DHHS) (see the Bibliography at the end of this chapter). According to the DHHS, the number of complaints filed by patients grew from fewer than 6600 in 2004 to more than 8100 in 2007. This increase may reflect patients' increased awareness of their rights as well as broader regulations that took effect during that time. All HIPAA complaints made by a patient, as soon as they become known to the practice, should be documented and filed with the privacy official. An example of an incident report is seen in Figure 3-4.

Figure 3-4
An example of an incident report.

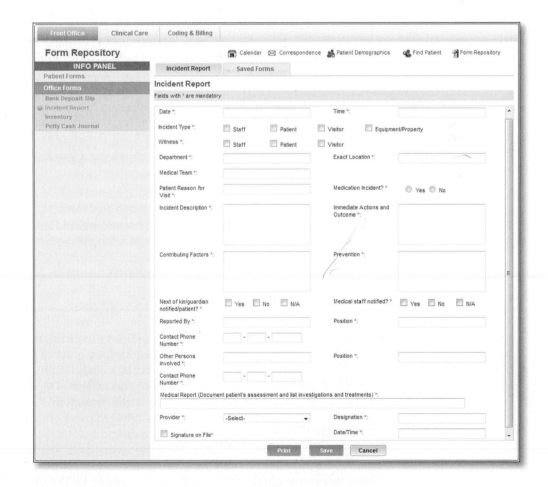

Ellen does not have the right to file a lawsuit against a covered entity for violating her rights under HIPAA. However, the provider is subject to civil penalties such as fines if found to be in violation. The process followed by the OCR when a patient lodges a complaint is shown in Figure 3-5.

Figure 3-5
The OCR complaint
process.

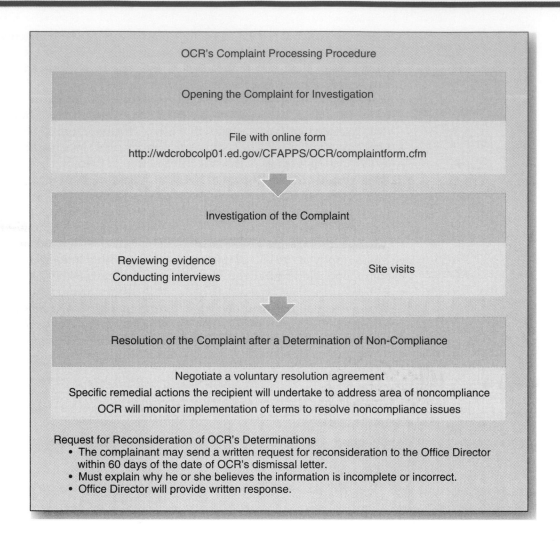

OCR's Complaint Processing Procedure

Opening the Complaint for Investigation

File with online form
http://wdcrobcolp01.ed.gov/CFAPPS/OCR/complaintform.cfm

Investigation of the Complaint

Reviewing evidence
Conducting interviews   Site visits

Resolution of the Complaint after a Determination of Non-Compliance

Negotiate a voluntary resolution agreement
Specific remedial actions the recipient will undertake to address area of noncompliance
OCR will monitor implementation of terms to resolve noncompliance issues

Request for Reconsideration of OCR's Determinations
- The complainant may send a written request for reconsideration to the Office Director within 60 days of the date of OCR's dismissal letter.
- Must explain why he or she believes the information is incomplete or incorrect.
- Office Director will provide written response.

After referring Tamara to the government's HIPAA website, Tamara agreed to release Ellen's records and apologized for her misunderstanding. In fact, as the privacy and security officer for the practice, Tamara has organized a lunchtime brown-bag refresher session on HIPAA for everyone on the staff.

OTHER SECURITY INITIATIVES

Along with the HIPAA regulations, other organizations and committees are trying to promote the use of secure EHR systems. The federal government's Office of the National Coordinator (ONC) for Health Information Technology, part of DHHS, released its Consolidated Health Informatics (CHI) initiative in 2003. The initiative is a collaborative effort involving about 20 federal agencies, including the DHHS, Department of Defense, and Department of Veterans Affairs. It aims to provide consistent standards for health information interoperability, terminology, and messaging to promote the electronic exchange of clinical information within the federal government.

The HITECH Act, part of the American Recovery and Reinvestment Act (ARRA) of 2009, details incentive for the adoption of health information technology as a means of accelerating its meaningful implementation. In addition, HITECH details security elements that work to enforce penalties and require breach of data notifications for facilities. Meaningful use programs are discussed in more detail in Chapter 4.

In addition, the Certification Commission for Healthcare Information Technology (CCHIT) is a cooperative coalition of leading healthcare industry organizations that promotes the adoption of interoperable EHR systems by healthcare facilities (see Chapter 1).

Although CCHIT is a private, not-for-profit effort, DHHS has contracted with CCHIT to accelerate certification in certain areas, including the following:

- EHR systems for office-based ambulatory care providers and specialists
- Inpatient EHR systems
- Health networks that exchange EHR data
- EHR systems within specific populations (such as behavioral health) in a range of care settings (including long-term care)

ACCESS TO PROTECTED HEALTH INFORMATION

As the United States converts to using EHR systems, it's critical for Americans to have confidence that their health information will not be exploited, misused, or accessed inappropriately. However, scandals like the Living Social data breach and the Target department store compromise of bank card information occurring in December 2013 have consumers on alert. Americans are becoming increasingly uncomfortable with the idea of having external entities collect and access—sometimes even package and sell—their personal information.

When it comes to the confidentiality, privacy, and security of patient records, it seems that knowledge is power—or at least reassurance. A survey of more than 1400 patients in Massachusetts who were using an EHR with email and online patient access features found that those with more education were less likely to be concerned about security and confidentiality.

A British study by Pyper and colleagues, this one also centering on an EHR system that allowed patients to access their own files, found that patients had less apprehension after using the system. Nearly half of the study participants felt uneasy about the security of their files before viewing them, but the figure dropped to only about 40% afterward.

The idea of security rests on the notion that certain parties have permission to view private medical information, whereas others are prohibited from doing so. So, who does have legal access to patients' records and in what circumstances?

Financial Institutions

In 1999 a federal law called the Financial Services Modernization Act went into effect. This law allows financial institutions—banks, securities firms, insurance companies, insurance agencies, thrifts, credit unions, mortgage brokers, finance companies, check cashers, and others—to join forces and operate as a single entity.

Medical information, such as payments made to a pharmacy or medical practice, can be shared freely within these so-called financial supermarkets and can be sold to outside third parties unless the account holder objects. The law does require companies to disclose their privacy practices and to allow customers to opt out of such disclosures. However, unless a person opts out, his or her medical information could pass into the hands of a third party, such as a retailer or direct-marketing firm. Remember, only healthcare institutions are subject to HIPAA. Financial institutions—with the exception of health insurance companies and other covered entities (see following)—are exempt.

✔ SECURITY CHECKPOINT 3-1

Medical Privacy Goes Offshore

This very moment, workers in New Delhi may be transcribing court proceedings related to an obstetric malpractice case in Detroit, answering a call from a patient in Denver who wants to know whether his insurance covers smoking cessation, and entering payment information for a 90-day prescription for birth control pills given to a young woman in Dallas.

The Financial Services Modernization Act does not prohibit financial institutions from sharing medical information with service providers, such as companies with which they contract to process accounting transactions and operate customer call centers. Financial companies that operate in the United States routinely outsource these functions to low-wage foreign workers, a practice known as *offshoring*. The work is sent to nations with large English-speaking populations, such as India, Sri Lanka, the Philippines, and Hong Kong.

These offshore workers may be asked to process personal financial and medical data, such as your name, Social Security number, account numbers, and diagnosis codes. Court transcription of medical cases and general medical transcription jobs are often sent offshore as well. The data are occasionally used for fraudulent purposes, such as medical identity theft involving fraudulent claims submission. In addition, a dishonest offshore worker may sell the information to criminals operating in the United States or may share it with a subcontractor who does so.

People who are harmed, financially or otherwise, by such misuse of their personal data have little recourse because these workers are not U.S. citizens, operate outside our borders, and thus are not governed by U.S. law. Legislators are debating ways of closing this gap in HIPAA privacy protection, a loophole that wasn't anticipated when the law was passed. Companies operating in countries that are part of the European Union (EU) have solved the problem by agreeing to send private data only to so-called safe harbor countries—those that have strong, enforceable privacy protections. Because few countries have privacy policies equivalent to those of the EU nations, fewer EU companies have turned to offshoring as a way of meeting their account management needs.

Alarm over offshoring medical information may be an overreaction, however. First, companies that handle offshore transcription, accounting, call centers, and other functions have a great deal at stake and can't prosper if they handle sensitive information carelessly. Consequently, they often follow stringent internal security procedures. Second, many Americans actually feel safer having highly personal medical data handled by people on another continent than by employees who may be in the next town or city. And finally, most foreign workers, like working folks in the United States, are just doing their jobs. They're honest, hardworking people who have no intention of misusing the information—nor any interest at all in our hemorrhoids and hammertoes.

Insurance Companies

As mentioned, an insurance company is an example of a covered entity—that is, any health-care entity that submits claims electronically, such as a medical office, hospital, nursing home, pharmacy, physical therapist, or clearinghouse. Covered entities must comply with all HIPAA standards, but patients must agree to permit insurance companies to access their records for purposes of claims submission and reimbursement and determination of insurability.

Government Agencies

The U.S. government has the right to see a patient's EHR without authorization in many circumstances. As discussed earlier when we met Michael and Ed, public health data are reported anonymously or confidentially for the purposes of tracking the incidence and spread of certain diseases. Other examples of government officials or agencies generally exempt from the HIPAA Privacy Rule include military healthcare plans, workers' compensation, correctional institutions, law enforcement officials, medical examiners, the FDA, and national security or intelligence officials, as required by the Patriot Act. A patient's records may even be reviewed by the DHHS during the course of investigating a privacy complaint.

CRITICAL THINKING EXERCISE 3-5

Two state troopers have just burst into your medical office demanding immediate help in tracking down a prisoner on the run. They believe the man may be responsible for an area carjacking, and they have a written request for a description of any distinguishing physical characteristics, such as scars and tattoos. The EHR reveals that the man has a large heart on his upper arm with the name "Pookie" written inside it. However, the officers don't have a warrant for the information. Can you give it to them? Does it matter whether the fugitive has committed a violent or a nonviolent offense?

Consumer Reporting Agencies

Most of us are aware that our credit is tracked by three major credit reporting agencies so that when we apply for a mortgage, car loan, credit card, or another form of credit, potential lenders can check our payment history before deciding whether to approve the loan. What we may not know is that **consumer reporting agencies** exist for other purposes, such as tenant reports for landlords, homeowners' and vehicle insurance claims reports, and employment background screening reports. Life, health, disability, and long-term care insurers rely on information from consumer reporting agencies to find out about patients' health and prescription drug histories. In addition, insurers are investigating the viability of databases to collect results from patients' laboratory tests, imaging studies, and pathology reports.

These so-called downstream agencies claim to release information only with the patient's **consent,** yet the companies are not subject to HIPAA regulations. Proposed legislation would allow federal regulators to audit the companies and to impose fines for privacy violations. In addition, consumer reporting agencies are subject to the Fair Credit Reporting Act (FCRA), which is intended to protect consumer privacy and to ensure the accuracy of information supplied by consumer reporting agencies. When an insurer takes an **adverse action**—that is, the denial or termination of insurance or a rate increase—based on information obtained from a **consumer reporting agency,** the insurer must send a notice informing the consumer of the decision and explaining the consumer's right to request a free copy of the report in question within 60 days. However, the insurer need not explain the specific reasons for its decision.

Before obtaining medical information from an EHR, health insurers or others who wish to view it must obtain the patient's consent, which might be done in a recorded telephone statement, by email, or with a signed hard copy. Failing to do so may prompt legal action from individuals, states, or federal agencies. The Federal Trade Commission (FTC) regulates compliance with the FCRA, and patients may contact the agency for information about the law or to file a complaint. (See the Bibliography at the end of this chapter.)

Medical Information Bureau

MIB, Inc., (MIB), known until recently as the Medical Information Bureau, is a nonprofit industry group and consumer reporting agency that maintains a database of medical information exchanged by the life, health, and disability insurers that make up its membership. You might think of it as an extensive electronic lending library where members drop by to swap information about patients' health histories. MIB saves its 470 member companies an estimated $1 billion per year by detecting and deterring fraudulent insurance claims. This savings is passed on to consumers, at least in part, in the form of lower health insurance premiums.

If a person has never been seriously injured or ill and has never made a health insurance claim, that person will not have an MIB file, just as there would be no credit report if the person has never taken out a loan or received credit of any kind. MIB reports that only about 20% of Americans have files, although this figure has not been independently confirmed.

Insurance companies are in the business of prediction, and the more information they have, the more accurate those predictions are likely to be. MIB collects any information that might have a bearing on how healthy a patient is likely to be and how long he or she is likely to live, such as the following:

- Acute and chronic illnesses
- Injuries
- Medical tests performed, the reasons the tests were ordered, and the results
- Modifiable risk factors, such as smoking, overweight, and obesity
- Lifestyle risk factors, such as gambling habits
- Substance abuse, including alcohol dependence, use of illegal drugs, and abuse of prescription drugs
- Hazardous occupations and pastimes, such as skydiving, flying private aircraft, and traveling to dangerous parts of the world
- Motor vehicle reports indicating poor driving skills and thus a likelihood of future accidents

Prescription Database Tools

Life insurance companies and other underwriters also rely on patients' prescription drug histories to make insurability decisions. About 200 million Americans' pharmacy purchases have been recorded in the files of Intelliscript or MedPoint, consumer reporting agencies that maintain databases of prescription purchasing histories. The companies sell these prescription profiles to insurance companies for about $15 each, saving insurers the time and expense of trying to retrieve the information from patients' physicians. The files are updated daily, and records stretch back 5 years.

Not only do these profiles tell insurers how much a patient's prescription drug costs are likely to be, they also reveal a great deal about a patient's health. A young woman receiving hydroxychloroquine (Plaquenil) and prednisone, for example, probably has lupus or a similar autoimmune disorder even if her EHR does not reveal that diagnosis directly. However, the prescription records can be misleading because so many drugs are prescribed for **off-label indications**—that is, for uses other than those for which the FDA has approved the drug. For instance, a person may be prescribed gabapentin (Neurontin) to treat neuropathic (nerve) pain. An insurance adjuster reviewing the file may presume that the person has been prescribed the drug for its primary indication, which is the treatment of epilepsy. However, combined with information from MIB, which comes directly from the patient's EHR, a more accurate diagnostic picture tends to emerge.

Like the credit reporting bureaus, which crunch the numbers from several sources in order to determine an overall credit score, the prescription database tools analyze the data in each patient's file to assign a risk score. This actual score is compared with an expected risk score to determine whether the patient is likely to be more or less expensive than most patients of the same gender and age.

Schools

Records of children's visits to the school nurse are covered by the Family Educational Rights and Privacy Act rather than by the HIPAA Privacy Rule.

Employers

Group health plans that cover 50 or more employees are subject to HIPAA, but the employer still has the right to know whether an employee is enrolled in the plan and has the right to review a summary of each employee's healthcare expenses. Self-insurance plans, on-site health promotion clinics and wellness centers, and other arrangements are considered hybrid entities and are subject to special privacy rules that generally offer patients less privacy protection. In most states, employers may ask employees to authorize disclosure of information in their EHR systems. This request may be made during the hiring process, when the employee is asked to authorize a complete background check, or it might occur during an orientation session. If employees are signing multiple documents, they may not even realize they have waived their right to the privacy of their EHR. (Patients should check the DHHS website for specific information.) Employers must also abide by Equal Employment Opportunity Commission (EEOC) regulations and by the provisions of the Americans with Disabilities Act (ADA) (see the Bibliography at the end of this chapter).

Family and Friends

Disclosure to family and friends is the source of more misunderstanding than perhaps any other area of HIPAA regulations. It is not true that a healthcare professional cannot speak to a patient's family or friends about his or her condition. The HIPAA Privacy Rule says that a provider or other covered entity may discuss IIHI with family members, close friends, or anyone else the patient specifies in order to inform them of the patient's general condition, location, or death, or to involve them in the patient's care, as long as the patient doesn't object.

If the patient is not available or is incapacitated and it can be reasonably inferred that the patient wouldn't object, the provider can disclose IIHI directly relevant to the patient's care if he or she believes it's in the patient's best interest to do so. A covered entity is also allowed to let another person pick up prescriptions, magnetic resonance imaging (MRI) films, and medical equipment, such as glucose meters and catheters.

Internet Communities

Most of us don't give a second thought to the medical information we disclose via a Facebook post or our latest tweet about going to the physician; these open web pages even link to our personal information, photographs, and physical location. Patients should review the privacy policies of every site that asks for personal information. Many sites actually capture, store, and even sell such information without patients' knowledge. Third parties have ever more financial incentive to collect, sell, and swap such information, which may make its way back to the EHR and subsequently to insurance companies, marketers, and others. Patients shouldn't necessarily refrain from posting something they do not necessarily want everyone in the world to see; they should just be aware that what they say may—and probably will—leave the page, especially if they offer identifying details about themselves.

Researchers

The American Medical Informatics Association lists research as an important **secondary use** of healthcare information—an application that is not directly related to patient care—that will be facilitated by a nationally interoperable system of records. Researchers are permitted to access patients' EHR systems if they have approval from their own educational institutions to do so. Most patients don't mind this kind of disclosure. Many surveys find that most American adults would release their health information to researchers with the caveat that any personally identifying details be omitted.

Direct Marketing Firms

Direct marketing is simply another term for what most of us call junk mail or spam. The American Civil Liberties Union (ACLU) and others worry that information in EHR systems may be disclosed for the purpose of what it calls "invasive direct marketing to patients by competitors." Earlier in this chapter you met Ellen, who has MS and has decided to take a more active role in her healthcare. Her EHR reveals that she's taking Avonex, known generically as interferon beta 1a. Under certain circumstances, the pharmaceutical company that makes Rebif, a competing interferon 1a drug, could gain access to her EHR to get this information and then market its own product directly to Ellen. The HIPAA Privacy Rule prohibits disclosure of IIHI from patients' EHR systems unless the communication occurs face to face or the direct marketer offers "a gift of nominal value." This second exception constitutes a rather large loophole. However, covered entities are prohibited from selling lists of patients or plan participants.

CRITICAL THINKING EXERCISE 3-6

You work in a practice with five gynecologists and a nurse practitioner. The office has just used its new EHR system to determine which of its female patients ages 40 and older have not yet had a mammogram or have not done so within the past year, and you and your staff have been asked to contact those patients. The patient's husband answers when you reach the third name on the list. What, if anything, can you tell him without violating your patient's privacy rights under HIPAA? Would it be better just to hang up?

HOW PATIENTS CAN PROTECT THEIR HEALTH INFORMATION

Patients are right to take an interest in protecting the integrity of their health information, which may be compromised by careless disposal or handling of records, lax security policies, and other breaches. Third parties who gain authorized or unauthorized access to a patient's health information can use it against the patient to discriminate in hiring or promotion, to reject an insurance application, to prevail in a legal proceeding, or simply to cause deliberate embarrassment. The following Security Checkpoint describes some unusually careless or devious ways in which security may be compromised.

✔ SECURITY CHECKPOINT 3-2

Top 10 Most Creative Explanations for Privacy Breaches

We've all heard of the hacker living in his parents' basement who breaks into a patient database, and we know about the occasional stolen laptop that contains thousands of patient files. But sensitive medical information has been discarded, lost, or stolen from both paper and digital files in much more imaginative ways and for much more curious or unscrupulous reasons. Our Top 10 list describes 10 privacy or security breaches that have been documented since HIPAA was enacted. The list may have a certain entertainment value, but there's a serious message just beneath the surface: Protect patients' information vigilantly, because someone is likely to want to take advantage of it if you don't.

10. **Attempted blackmail.** In a payment dispute with the Veterans Administration, an offshore contractor threatened to disclose the health information of tens of thousands of veterans. In a similar dispute with the University of California–San Francisco Medical Center, a transcriptionist in Pakistan threatened to post EHR systems on the Internet. Although he was persuaded not to do so, the medical center was unable to confirm that he had destroyed the files as requested.

9. **Winning a quarrel.** In the midst of a restructuring, whistleblowers within the Washington, D.C., emergency medical services division leaked medical information about several patients in an effort to prove their contention that the delivery of care by firefighter-paramedics was substandard. The physician who served as quality assurance director was fired over the incident.

8. **Guaranteeing future insurability.** A woman in New England admitted to a *New York Times* reporter that she had lifted page after page from her own paper medical chart after seeing that her physician had noted repeatedly that she was at risk for Huntington's disease, a fatal genetic condition from which the woman's mother had died. The woman did not know whether she had the disease but feared that neither she nor her children would be eligible for affordable health insurance if such a grave risk became known to the insurance companies. The pilfering patient was never caught.

7. **Dumpster ditching.** An intrepid local news team in Michigan "surveyed" Dumpsters behind area medical practices and discovered that using a paper shredder was apparently just too much of a hassle for staff members. Half of the practices had tossed intact files or other documents, many containing names, Social Security numbers, and potentially embarrassing treatment information, right into the trash. In a similar exposé, CVS and Walgreen's pharmacies in Houston were found to be dumping patients' private health information into their Dumpsters.

6. **Hitting "Reply All"—Oops!** A statistician working for Florida's Palm Beach County Health Department accidentally sent an email attachment containing the names of thousands of HIV/AIDS patients to 800 other county employees.

5. **Ambulance chasing.** In Nassau County, New York, the district attorney's office revealed that certain hospital employees had been caught accepting payola from corrupt attorneys and medical clinics for disclosing the identities of accident victims. The patients were then contacted by the lawyers or clinic staff and asked to participate in schemes involving fraudulent insurance claims.

4. **Sharing a laugh at the patient's expense.** According to the *New York Daily News*, a Brooklyn, New York, EMT was suspended without pay after a colleague reported he had scanned and emailed the medical records of patients who had been injured in circumstances that the

EMT considered to be humorous. The records contained identifying details about patients as well as a description of their injuries.

3. **Protecting the environment.** An environmentally conscious San Joaquin County employee placed a box of unshredded mental health records out for curbside recycling at his home in Stockton, California. He was fired after being ratted out by a neighbor.

2. **Protecting the public.** In Pennsylvania, inmates' mental health records are considered public property under the state's "Right to Know" law.

1. **Tracking the sniffles.** The American Civil Liberties Union contends that forcing customers to show identification and sign a log in order to purchase pseudoephedrine-containing cold medicine (such as Sudafed), which in large quantities is used to produce methamphetamine, could unfairly place under suspicion anyone who is a regular user. These products used to be available over the counter, but in at least 35 states, customers must now purchase them at a pharmacy counter, where their identities are recorded. In Oregon, a prescription is now required to purchase pseudoephedrine.

Besides guarding against such outcomes, patients should stay vigilant to make sure their records are free of inaccuracies caused by simple human error. Some inaccuracies could affect a patient's health, such as incorrect dates or frequencies of disease recurrences or even incorrect sites of amputation.

Ellen plans to take the following steps recommended by medical privacy advocates to make sure her medical information stays within her control:

- **Review medical, dental, and prescription drug records for accuracy.** Ellen requested copies of her files from MIB, IntelliScript, and MedPoint (see the Bibliography at the end of this chapter for contact information). She also requested copies of her records from the local hospital at which she has had several surgeries and from her neurologist, ophthalmologist, gastroenterologist, general practitioner, and dentist. She reviewed them for accuracy and discovered a transcription error in one of them, showing her prescription for Dantrolene, a muscle relaxant, as Diprolene, a skin cream prescribed to patients with psoriasis. She requested an amendment, which was made (in compliance with HIPAA) within 60 days.

- **Request a disclosure log.** Ellen wanted to know who had accessed her records, so she requested an accounting of disclosures from her physician. The HIPAA Privacy Rule requires covered entities to account for disclosures of IIHI from a patient's EHR for purposes other than treatment, payment, healthcare operations, national security or intelligence, and law enforcement, and in certain other limited circumstances.

- **Request restrictions on disclosure of sensitive information.** Patients have the right to ask a covered entity to restrict the disclosure of health information for payment purposes. The covered entity is not required to approve the request, but if it does it then has an obligation to honor the restriction. Ellen, for instance, is insured through her husband's group plan. If she wished to do so, she could ask her provider and insurance company not to disclose her IIHI to her husband even in the course of answering his payment questions.

- **Ask to receive correspondence at alternative locations.** The Privacy Rule also requires covered entities to accommodate patients who wish to receive correspondence or other communications containing IIHI, such as telephone messages, by alternative means or at alternative locations. This information is documented under the HIPAA folder of the electronic patient record. For example, Ellen has asked that all messages be left on her cell phone. The covered entity may ask, in return, that the patient inform them of where bills should be sent and who will take responsibility for paying them.

- **Pay out of pocket.** Ellen has decided to seek help for depression, but she and her husband believe it's best to pay cash for the visits. Some healthcare folks call this "staying off the grid"—that is, paying directly for certain services, such as addiction counseling, rather than submitting the bills for insurance reimbursement and thus having private information disclosed to an insurer or other third party.

- **Opt for online versus paper statements and read them carefully.** Most Americans believe that some of their private health information or that of a loved one has been lost or stolen from a medical practice, healthcare institution, insurance company, employer, or government agency (such as Medicare) at one time or another. Seventy percent of Americans believe that electronic records are more likely to be lost or stolen or that paper and electronic records are subject to loss or theft about equally. This is a misconception. When it comes to identity theft, most criminals still work the old-fashioned way—by swiping mail right out of your mailbox. Remember, most statements that are printed and mailed are part of a database at the insurance company or provider network. So when a patient receives paper statements, thieves have two chances to steal the personal information. But a database is more secure than an unlocked mailbox, hands down.

Ellen used to receive paper statements from most of her physicians, declining to switch to electronic statements even when urged to do so. She also used to throw away or shred the statements without looking at them if she had a zero balance. Now she's made the switch to emailed statements. When a link to a new statement arrives in her in-box, she clicks on it and reads the Explanation of Benefits section carefully, regardless of whether she owes the provider. She also plans to check her regular credit report at least once a year to look for any medical debts that she did not incur.

EHR EXERCISE 3-4:   PATIENT RECORD ACCESS REQUEST

*Complete the following exercise in the EHR Exercises environment of SimChart for the Medical Office.

Mr. Ken Thomas (10-25-1961) of Larkin Avenue would like to view the contents of his record to confirm no incorrect information has been documented. He has requested an appointment with the privacy officer who has instructed him to complete a Patient Record Access Request form. Mr. Thomas is interested specifically in Progress Notes and Hospitalizations from March 2009 to December 2013. Document the expiration date as 30 days from today.

1. Select the Patient Record Access Request from the left info panel of the Form Repository and use the Patient Search button to link the document to the patient record before proceeding.

2. Fill in the blank text fields and save the completed document to the patient record using the Save to Patient Record button.

CHAPTER SUMMARY

- Medical privacy is the right to decide when, how much, and with whom health information can be shared. Patients may have the expectation that this right exists, but privacy is a legal concept subject to specific exceptions and limitations.
- The original impetus for passage of HIPAA was to protect the insurability of patients with preexisting conditions as they switched insurers. However, the law has since been greatly expanded in an effort to ensure patient privacy and protect the security of electronic health information.
- Administrative safeguards outlined by the HIPAA Security Rule include risk analysis, risk management, sanctions (penalties), and information system activity review. A security officer must be assigned to oversee the development and implementation of security policies, education, practices, and procedures.
- The record of a user's electronic path through the EHR system is called an audit trail.
- Under HIPAA, patients have the right to view or receive copies of their health record, request corrections, receive a notice of privacy practices, opt out of sharing certain information with certain people, have certain information withheld from certain third parties, receive a list of disclosures of their health information, and file a complaint.
- CHI is an initiative that aims to establish consistent standards for health information interoperability, terminology, and messaging in order to promote the electronic

exchange of clinical information within the federal government. CCHIT is a private-sector, cooperative coalition of leading healthcare industry organizations that promotes the adoption of interoperable EHR systems by healthcare facilities.

- Many interested parties may have access to an employee's health information, including financial companies, insurers, public health agencies, law enforcement officials, consumer reporting agencies, schools, employers, family and friends, Internet communities, researchers, and direct marketing firms.

- Consumer reporting agencies sell or cooperatively exchange consumer information and history in areas such as credit and health. They include MIB, Inc., formerly known as the Medical Information Bureau, and for-profit prescription database tools such as Intelliscript and MedPoint.

- Patients can protect the privacy and integrity of the information in their EHR systems by reviewing their records, requesting a disclosure log, placing restrictions on whom they'd like the provider to share information with, and reviewing their statements carefully even when they owe no money.

CHAPTER REVIEW ACTIVITIES

Key Terms Review

Match the following key terms with their definitions.

1. Protected health information (PHI)
2. Covered entities
3. Laws
4. Password
5. Privacy
6. Confidentiality
7. Consent
8. Anonymity
9. Disclosure
10. Authentication
11. Individually identifiable health information (IIHI)
12. Secondary use
13. Minimum necessary standard
14. Ethics
15. Consumer reporting agency

a. The patient's right and expectation that individually identifiable health information will be kept private

b. Giving access to, releasing, or transferring health information to another person or entity

c. Individually identifiable health information that is stored, maintained, or transmitted electronically

d. Healthcare providers, health plans, and healthcare clearinghouses that transmit claims electronically

e. An agency that sells or cooperatively exchanges consumer information and history in areas such as credit and healthcare

f. The patient's right to have private health data collected in such a way that it can never be linked to him or her

g. A character sequence used to prevent unauthorized access to patient information contained in secure electronic files

h. The process of determining whether the person attempting to access a given network or EHR system is authorized to do so

i. Formal, enforceable rules and policies based on community standards of conduct

j. The patient's freedom to determine when, how much, and under what circumstances his or her medical information may be disclosed

k. A key provision of the HIPAA Privacy Rule requiring that disclosures include no more than the amount of information necessary to accomplish a given purpose

l. Permission given to a covered entity for uses and disclosures of protected health information for treatment, payment, and healthcare operations

m. A use of health information for a business activity or other purpose that is not directly related to patient care

n. Health information that clearly identifies an individual patient or could reasonably be used to identify the patient

o. Rules and standards of conduct that govern professional behavior and arise from our shared understanding of morality

True/False

Indicate whether the statement is true or false.

1. _____When a patient requests confidentiality regarding particular test results or diagnoses, the provider is obligated to hold that information in confidence.

2. _____Covered entities—healthcare providers, health plans, and healthcare clearinghouses—are subject to the HIPAA Privacy Rule.

3. _____The HIPAA Security Rule outlines the administrative, physical, and technologic measures covered entities must take in order to implement and comply with the HIPAA Privacy Rule.

4. _____HITECH requires that physician offices begin implementing an EHR immediately.

5. _____A computer can verify that a password is valid but cannot authenticate that the person using the password is authorized to do so.

6. _____A screensaver is used to limit the view of patient information on a computer screen while the user is away from his or her desk.

7. _____If erroneous information is found in a file, it can be removed at the patient's request.

8. _____HIPAA prohibits financial institutions from obtaining medical information.

9. _____A healthcare professional may speak to a patient's family or friends about the patient's general condition and location as long as the patient doesn't object or, if the patient is incapacitated, it can reasonably be inferred that he or she wouldn't object.

Workplace Applications

Using the knowledge you obtained from the chapter, provide narrative answers to the following cases.

1. You are the privacy officer for your practice, and a new employee complains to you about the excessive HIPAA training she is enduring. What can you tell this employee about why such training is necessary?

2. As you're walking toward the lunchroom, you pass a computer that has a patient's health information displayed from the EHR. You are able to clearly see a list of the patient's medications. What safety measures can the office take to prevent such unintentional disclosure of PHI?

3. Juliette Zimmerman is the volunteer coach of the high school cheerleading team. The team has earned a spot at nationals, but one of her flyers is injured and will not be able to participate. Juliette has just given an interview to a local reporter in which she made mention of this, including the girl's name. Juliette's husband, a physician, tells her that she has violated HIPAA. Is he correct?

4. You work in a psychiatry practice, and many of your patients with health insurance prefer to pay cash to protect their privacy. If a patient does submit a mental health claim, in what circumstances might that information be disclosed to a third party without the patient's authorization? How might this practice of paying "off the grid" affect public mental health services?

5. You work in a urology practice, and a 51-year-old married patient, Mr. Ratner, undergoes a vasectomy because he does not wish to have any more children. He confides to the physician that he's concerned his mistress may become pregnant. He has the procedure performed while his wife is out of town, and he requests that information about the vasectomy not be disclosed to her under any circumstances. Does Mrs. Ratner have the right to know that her husband has had a vasectomy? Does Mr. Ratner's physician or his staff have a right or an obligation to tell her? If Mrs. Ratner is also a patient in the practice, does that change your answer?

6. Chase Murray Jr. (04-07-1993) is new to the Walden-Martin office. Part of the new patient procedures is to provide the patient with a copy of the NPP and patient's bill of rights. Use SCMO to print and save a copy of these documents to Chase's record.

EHR in Review

Complete the following exercises based on content previously covered in Chapters 1 and 2.

1. Truong Tran (05-30-1991) has picked up another insurance plan. MetLife insurance will now be his secondary insurance payer; Aetna will still remain as primary. Add this new insurance carrier to Truong's record.
   MetLife Insurance
   Policy ID Number: XXT65667

Group Number: PA57

Claims Address: 1234 Insurance Avenue, Anytown, AL 12345

Claim Phone Number: 800-877-0909

*Truong is the Policy Holder of this secondary insurance

2. Name the eight core functions of an EHR.

3. Define clinical decision support (CDS) tools and give one example of how they are used.

BIBLIOGRAPHY

Adams, W. L. (2009). *Coding and reimbursement: A simplified approach* (3rd ed.). St. Louis: Elsevier.

Apse, K. A., Biesecker B. B., Giardello, F. M., et al. (2004). Perceptions of genetic discrimination among at-risk relatives of colorectal cancer patients. *Genetics in Medicine*, 6, 510–516.

Becklin, K. J. (2006). *Medical office procedures* (6th ed.). New York: McGraw-Hill.

Department of Health and Human Services, Centers for Medicare and Medicaid. *HIPAA security series*. Available at www.cms.hhs.gov/EducationMaterials/04_SecurityMaterials.asp. Accessed 18.12.08.

Department of Health and Human Services, Office of Civil Rights. *Compliance and enforcement health information privacy complaints received by calendar year*. Available at www.hhs.gov/ocr/privacy/enforcement/data/complaintsyear.html. Accessed 20.12.08.

Department of Health and Human Services, Office of Civil Rights. *HIT certification*. Available at www.hhs.gov/healthit/certification/cchit. Accessed 20.12.08.

Department of Health and Human Services, Office of the Secretary. (2002). *Federal Register: Standards for privacy of individually identifiable health information, part V; Final rule*. (Vol. 67 157 August 14). Available at www.hhs.gov/ocr/hipaa/privrulepd.pdf. Accessed 17.12.08.

Fordney, M. T. (2006). *Insurance handbook for the medical office* (9th ed.). St. Louis: Elsevier.

Harmon, A. (2008). Congress passes bill to bar bias based on genes. *The New York Times*, May 2.

Harris Interactive. (2007). *The Harris Poll*. #27, March 26.

Harris Interactive. (2008). *The Harris Poll*. #74, July 15.

Hassol, J., Walker, J. M., Kidder, D., et al. (2004). Patient experiences and attitudes about access to a patient electronic health care record and linked web messaging. *Journal of the American Medical Informatics Association*, 11, (6), 505–513.

Health Privacy Project. (2007). Health privacy stories. March 5. Available at www.healthprivacy.org/usr_doc/Privacystories.pdf. Accessed 09.12.08.

The Johns Hopkins Genetics and Public Policy Center. (2007). U.S. public opinion on uses of genetic information and genetic discrimination, April 24. Available at http://www.dnapolicy.org/resources/GINAPublic_Opinion_Genetic_Information_Discrimination.pdf. Accessed 02.24.14.

Kaufman, D. J., Murphy, J., Scott, J., et al. (2008). Subjects matter: A survey of public opinions about a large cohort study. *Genetics in Medicine*, 10, 831–839.

Nakashima, E. (2008). Prescription data used to assess consumers: Records aid insurers but prompt privacy concerns. *Washington Post*, August 4.

Peel, D. C. (2007). *Privacy and confidentiality concerns in the nationwide health information network*. Institute for Behavioral Health Informatics: Plenary Keynote Address, October 26.

Pyper, C., Amery, J., Watson, M., et al. (2004). Patients' experiences when accessing their on-line electronic patient records in primary care. *The British Journal of General Practice*, 54, pp. 38-43.

Safran, C., Bloomrosen, M., Hammond, W. E., et al. (2006). Toward a national framework for the secondary use of health data. *American Medical Informatics Association*, September 14.

Stanley, J., Steinhardt, B. (2003). *Bigger monster, weaker chains: The growth of an American surveillance society*. ACLU Technology and Liberty Program, January. Available at www.aclu.org/FilesPDFs/aclu_report_bigger_monster_weaker_chains.pdf. Accessed 15.12.08.

University of Michigan. (2007). *C. S. Mott Children's Hospital national poll on children's health* Vol. 1.

chapter 4

Implementing Electronic Health Records

Chapter Outline

Commission on Accreditation of Allied Health Education Programs (CAAHEP) Competencies

1. Discuss applications of electronic technology in effective communication.
2. Discuss principles of using the electronic medical record (EMR).
3. Use office hardware and software to maintain office systems.

Chapter Objectives

1. Explain the considerations that must be addressed in planning a successful transition from paper charts to electronic health record (EHR) systems.
2. Develop a conversion plan for the EHR.
3. Explain the requirements of the Centers for Medicare & Medicaid Services (CMS) meaningful use program for eligible professionals.
4. Describe the information a practice should supply to each software vendor in its request for proposal document, and outline the information the practice should expect to receive from the vendors in return.

5. Give examples of the workflow processes that must be redesigned when an EHR system is implemented.

6. Outline the process of collecting and entering data from paper sources into the EHR.

7. Discuss common problems that may be encountered when information is transferred from paper charts to EHR systems.

8. Identify specific challenges that may arise in training to use a new EHR system.

9. Indicate how patients can be introduced to the new EHR system.

10. Specify the contingency plans that must be in place before an EHR is launched.

11. Discuss the EHR implementation process.

12. Explain how the success of an EHR can be measured after the transition period ends.

Key Terms

application service provider (ASP)   A company that provides online access to a software application; it requires a licensing agreement with the end-user. Application service provider arrangements allow the end-user to access software over the Internet and can be a less expensive alternative to purchasing a copy of the software and installing it on the user's local (on-site) server.

applications software (usually referred to simply as "application")   A program or suite of programs with word processing, graphics, database, spreadsheet, or other capabilities that is used to accomplish work-related tasks by the user.

client-server model   An architecture in which a powerful central computer serves a network of connected PCs or other workstations, called clients. The interface that allows the client and server to communicate (Windows or Linux, for example) resides on the client's computer. The software application and stored files (patients' records) reside on the server, which shares them when it receives a request from the client.

cloning   Copying and pasting notes from a patient's previous visit into the current progress note (also called "carrying forward") or pasting notes from one patient's record into the record of a patient with a similar diagnosis and presentation.

controlled vocabulary   A standardized list of preferred terms for medical diagnoses, findings, procedures, services, and treatments, along with machine-readable numeric codes that identify them. Examples include ICD diagnosis codes, CPT procedure codes, and NDC prescription codes.

data capture   The process of indirectly entering data into a system by recording (capturing) it electronically and converting it to machine-readable form. Examples of data capture methods include bar coding, voice recognition software, and structured templates.

go live   To become operational; the point at which the offline practice mode ends and real-world, online use begins. Often used in the phrase "go-live date."

hybrid   A medical office in which health records are stored and accessed in various formats—paper charts, EHR systems, and perhaps microfilm, microfiche, or other media.

legacy   A functional EHR system slated to be replaced with newer software.

organizational culture   The shared set of values, beliefs, and assumptions that governs the perceptions and interactions of the organization's members and guides their behavior and decision making.

preimplementation process   The process of training the staff and gathering the resources necessary to implement a conversion from a paper-based or legacy EHR to a new EHR system; the preparation phase that occurs before the go-live date.

records management   The systematic control of patient records, from creation through maintenance and storage.

request for proposal (RFP)   A formal written request sent to a shortlist of software vendors outlining the practice's needs, resources, time frame, and budget and requesting specific information about customer support, software features and proposed platform, tentative preimplementation plan, and estimated costs.

structured data entry   Use of mouse clicks, touch-screen commands, or simple keystroke combinations to enter data that conform to a controlled vocabulary; structured data entry helps practitioners input a large amount of information efficiently and is appropriate for describing typical signs, symptoms, and other straightforward clinical facts and findings.

template Predefined, customizable forms that facilitate structured data collection by offering the clinician a set of menus, check boxes, and other tools with which to enter data into progress notes, letters, and other EHR documents.

unstructured data entry Free data entry (as opposed to structured data entry using a controlled vocabulary) using direct keying, dictation, or transcription; unstructured data entry is needed to describe nuanced patient presentations and unique individual health histories.

virtual private network (VPN) A pathway that allows encrypted data to travel securely through an Internet connection to its destination, where it is unencrypted.

workflow A set of related tasks necessary to complete a step in a business process.

PLANNING FOR A SUCCESSFUL TRANSITION

A methodic approach seems to be the key to making a successful EHR transition. The first step in a well-planned transition is to assess the practice's readiness for the change. Some questions to consider include the following:

- What is the practice's motivation for making the change? What does it hope to achieve in making this change?
- Will the **organizational culture** support a technologic conversion and can it endure the frustrations and sacrifices associated with it?
- Are patients likely to support a migration from paper to digital charting?
- Does the practice have, or can it obtain at a reasonable cost, the necessary technologic and operational resources to make the switch?
- Does the practice have enough capital in reserve to stay afloat during a period of reduced productivity? Does it have enough cash on hand to purchase hardware, software or a software license, and training and information technology (IT) support?

CRITICAL THINKING EXERCISE 4-1

Do you think the practice in which you work is ready to cross the digital divide? If not, which of the areas just listed is likely to prove problematic? If you do not yet work in a medical practice, which factors do you think would most strongly influence readiness?

The **preimplementation process** itself offers a chance for the practice to examine these questions in depth. Even if it has already decided to go digital, assessing readiness will produce a useful inventory of strengths and weaknesses. The practice that enters this phase with some idea of what its soft spots are is already a step ahead.

A project manager or transition leader should be designated because a lack of clear direction can stall the conversion. Firm leadership is a key factor in the success of an EHR rollout. An unofficial champion or problem solver often emerges during the transition—a staff member or clinician with a special adeptness at using the EHR who becomes the "go to" person when wrinkles need to be ironed out or a workaround developed.

Although few studies have been published, the available evidence indicates the advantages of arranging prelaunch and rollout training, clearly assigning and delineating responsibilities, structuring and testing redesigned workflow processes, customizing documentation templates, collecting and entering data before the transition, and ensuring interoperability with key interfaced networks.

In this chapter we discuss these elements, direct you to some helpful resources, and offer some more detailed questions to consider as you plan the conversion at your office. Even if you've already left paper charts in the dust, reviewing these issues will help you adjust current procedures for optimal efficiency. You might even find ways of helping others who are in the process of going digital.

EASING THE TRANSITION 4-1

Will Social Networking Technology Allow Veteran EHR Users to Coach Novices Online?

We've all heard the cliché that it's not *what* you know, it's *who* you know. The phenomenon of social networking rests on this idea—which often turns out to be true. Most of us are familiar with social networking through online communities like LinkedIn, Facebook, and Twitter. The idea is to spin a web of business contacts and tap into other people's networks. This expanded network allows you to meet people to whom you might not otherwise have been introduced.

Social networks are also helpful in connecting those who share common interests or concerns—everyone from wine enthusiasts to language students, crime victims, and people living with Parkinson's. The common denominator among social networking sites is that people who know something share it with those who don't. The concept could work brilliantly for those planning to implement or who are learning to use an EHR. Those who have been through the process could share their knowledge and experience with those who are still working out the kinks.

BioMedExperts.com, the brainchild of Collexis Corporation, uses social networking technology to unite medical researchers in precisely this way. The site gives users free access to more than a million profiles of researchers in basic and applied science. The profiles are automatically generated, according to the company, by culling information from 6 million scientific publications, including 6500 research journals. Users can find their own profile, if one has been created, and customize it. Users can also view and communicate with their own network of coauthors, invite people to join their network, look for researchers with particular interests, and so on.

Although social networking is familiar to nearly every experienced computer user, its application to healthcare hasn't quite reached the tipping point, but it's catching on fast. Look for a community of EHR users to show up in your online neighborhood any day now.

DEVELOPING A CONVERSION PLAN

Many medical offices are convinced that converting from paper procedures to electronic practices is inevitable. The process is a little like quitting smoking—painful but necessary, with a big payoff when you finally succeed. Nevertheless, whether they've grudgingly accepted this conclusion or are eager to convert, they tend to delay the transition. Sometimes they simply don't know where to start.

To make the steps of the preimplementation process more concrete, let's look at how they might unfold in practice. Drs. Krutsch, Lymping, and Foosh have a small sports medicine office near Lake Placid, New York. A fourth physician, Dr. Idlewild, is semiretired and works remotely from his lakefront Adirondack cottage. He's available for consultation and, as a float-plane pilot, often visits the office to assist in treating patients with complex injuries.

The practice has a year-round clientele of serious amateur skiers, snowboarders, mountain bikers, speed skaters, ice climbers, and even the occasional luge pilot or dogsled racer. A seasonal group of tourists also keeps the practice busy, showing up with injuries typical of novices in most of the aforementioned sports. The physicians, who bill themselves as "The Moguls of Sports Medicine," or just "The Moguls" for short, have decided to convert to an EHR system.

Despite their nickname, The Moguls realize they don't run the show by themselves. They employ a full-time nurse practitioner, an office manager, and two medical assistants. They know from the experience of other users that all of their staff members' opinions must be represented during the prelaunch decision-making and planning phases. After all, each type of user will use the system in a different way. Having a good sense of all users' needs will ensure that the system they select has the right features and is properly customized. This will minimize the downtime caused by the transition.

CRITICAL THINKING EXERCISE 4-2

Cedars-Sinai Medical Center in Los Angeles offers an instructive example of an EHR system that worked as planned but nevertheless had to be withdrawn because it did not meet users' needs. The system's CPOE function included built-in alerts for dangerous drug interactions. These warnings could not be overridden even when the physician believed the potential benefit to the patient outweighed the risk. Dangerous delays occurred in delivering medications to critically ill patients, including children, as physicians tried to work around the automated system. How, specifically, could this situation have been avoided? What other kinds of problems might crop up when a system is too rigidly designed or is geared toward one kind of user rather than another?

The office manager at The Moguls, Meg Thatcher, was asked to take charge of the conversion plan. She scoured blogs and journal articles to look for helpful resources. She read published reports of other practices' transition experiences and CMS guidelines for meaningful use so that The Moguls could make the most out of their EHR adoption and avoid the most common mistakes (Table 4-1). She discussed relevant information at weekly staff meetings during several months of planning.

Table 4-1   *Pitfalls of EHR Transitions*

Problem	Effect	Prevention or Troubleshooting
Poorly designed software or lack of network server capacity	Security vulnerabilities, poor performance, implementation delays, crashes and downtime, undermining of confidence in system, lower productivity; need for expensive upgrades	Conduct accurate needs assessment, accounting for future growth of the practice; purchase more bandwidth or switch servers if necessary
Selection of complex hardware requiring advanced maintenance capabilities	Inability to support, maintain, or operate the EHR hardware lengthens downtime, increases repair costs, and weakens confidence in the system	A practice should install the simplest system that meets its needs, including any realistic expectation of expansion
Inadequate training, including hands-on support, during rollout	Launch delays, lower productivity during rollout, staff frustration, ineffective implementation, higher long-term training and implementation costs	Investigate training offered by software vendor before purchasing; set up mandatory training on a predetermined schedule; train before launch; set up a mentoring system or use social networking technology to coach staff
Poor leadership or lack of buy-in from staff or providers	Reluctance to participate in training; delayed launch; lower productivity during rollout; staff frustration and poor morale; ineffective implementation; higher costs; potential for project failure	Adequate training of project leader(s) and meticulous prelaunch planning; adequate staffing; reassignment of responsibilities if necessary
Underestimation of transition requirements	Delays; frustration; increased costs; project failure	Accurate analysis of the practice's needs and resources; thorough, meticulous planning; plan in place for quick recognition and redress of problems as they arise
Compromised patient care during launch and rollout	Patients could be harmed, causing pain, injury, or emotional distress; clinic is left vulnerable to legal action	Test runs and extensive prelaunch training, especially in critical areas such as prescription ordering and review of test results
Use of advanced CDS tools too soon	Confusion and frustration among clinicians already trying to master a new system; erosion of confidence in the system and in users' own abilities	Introduce advanced features gradually, as users' confidence increases
Insufficient funding	Delays during launch and rollout; incomplete implementation; lower productivity because software or hardware chosen does not meet the needs of the practice; possible implementation failure	Careful selection of software system and hardware support to maintain a balance between capacity and features versus cost

Meaningful Use Certification

As mentioned in Chapter 1, the Office of the National Coordinator for Health Information Technology (ONCHIT) has established requirements for EHR certification as part of the American

Recovery and Reinvestment Act (ARRA). EHR vendors are evaluated on a set of core and menu objective measures. The meaningful use (MU) incentive program is a payment incentive program made available for eligible professionals (EPs) or physicians who implement and use their EHR technology in a meaningful way. EPs can earn up to $44,000 throughout the course of this program, but their EHR usage must meet specific requirements. These are organized into three stages of core and menu objectives. The main goals of the MU program are:

- Improve quality, safety, and efficiency and reduce health disparities
- Engage patients and family
- Improve care coordination and population and public health
- Maintain privacy and security of patient health information

The MU program is divided into three parts. The goal was to allow a slow but meaningful implementation of electronic technology. In 2011–2012, stage 1 of MU was made available. This stage was referred to as data capture and sharing. Under the policy, providers must successfully complete stage 1 requirements before continuing to stage 2. Stage 2, advance clinical processes, is under way and will continue throughout 2014-2016. This stage builds on the established objectives to increase use and evaluation. For example, under stage 1 requirements, EPs are required to document demographics as structured data for more than 40% of patients. The stage 2 requirement increases that value to 50% of all patients. As these requirements have providers scrambling to get their data in order and new workflow underway, the implementation date for stage 3, improved outcomes, has been pushed back to 2017. It is hoped that this will give providers enough time to understand how their data monitoring is affecting patients and give EHR vendors enough time to be compliant under the strict stage 3 requirements expected to be announced.

Core Objectives

1. Use computerized provider order entry (CPOE) for medication orders directly entered.
2. Implement drug-drug and drug-allergy interaction checks.
3. Maintain an up-to-date problem list of current diagnoses.
4. Generate and transmit permissible prescriptions electronically.
5. Maintain active medication list.
6. Maintain active medication allergy list.
7. Record demographics (preferred language, gender, race, ethnicity, date of birth).
8. Record and chart vital signs (height, weight, blood pressure [BP], body mass index [BMI], growth charts).
9. Record smoking status.
10. Report ambulatory clinical quality measures.
11. Implement one clinical decision support (CDS) rule.
12. Provide patients with an electronic copy of their health information upon request.
13. Provide clinical summaries for patients for each office visit.
14. Protect electronic health information.
15. Stage 2 objective: Use secure electronic messaging to communicate with patients.

Menu Objectives

1. Implement drug formulary checks.
2. Incorporate clinical lab test results into the EHR as structured data.
3. Generate lists of patients by specific conditions to use for quality improvement.
4. Send patient reminders for preventive/follow-up care.
5. Provide patients with timely electronic access to their health information within 4 business days.
6. Identify patient-specific education resources and provide those resources to the patient.
7. Perform medication reconciliation.
8. Provide summary care record for transition or care or referral.
9. Submit electronic data to immunization registries.
10. Submit electronic syndromic surveillance data to public health agencies.

Additional Stage 2 Menu Objectives

11. Record electronic notes in patient records (progress notes).
12. Make imaging results accessible.
13. Record patient family health history as structured data.
14. Attain the capability to identify and report cancer cases to a state cancer registry.
15. Attain the capability to identify and report specific cases to a specialized registry (other than cancer).

SELECTING THE TYPE OF CONVERSION

Switching to an EHR system can be a long, exasperating process. A network of practices may spend as long as 5 years completing the preimplementation process. One of the first big decisions any medical practice must make is whether to switch completely to electronic **records management**—like going cold turkey, if you will, by giving up paper charts all at once—or to make an incremental (gradual) change. Another possibility is to become a **hybrid** office, in which existing patients' charts are kept on paper and only new patients are entered into the electronic database. A hybrid arrangement is essentially a very slow incremental conversion because eventually—although it will take years—existing patients will pass away, move, or switch practices, leaving only patients with electronic records. Some offices have already been using an EHR, usually an early-generation software system with limited functionality, and face the difficult task of converting a **legacy** EHR to a newer system.

EASING THE TRANSITION 4-2

Migrating from a Legacy EHR to a New System

When did you purchase your first cell phone, LCD TV, iPod, or GPS system? Were you willing to pony up a premium and take a chance that the bugs might not have been worked out yet? Or did you stand on the sidelines for a bit, waiting to see whether the hot new gadget would gain popularity?

Technology adoption forms a classic bell curve. Most users fall along the middle of the curve, embracing the new technology once the price has come down a bit and the product has been road tested by those more inclined to accept risk. We call these risk takers *early adopters*—the small percentage of users who are among the first to embrace a new technology. In healthcare, clinics affiliated with teaching hospitals have tended to be early adopters of EHR technology, perhaps because they're better funded and more innovative than an average private practice.

As the EHR systems in place at these clinics have matured, many practices have begun to switch to newer applications that offer greater functionality and increased efficiency. Zandieh and colleagues compared paper-to-EHR conversions with legacy EHR transitions and found that they present a unique set of considerations. First, the practice's reasons for upgrading to a new system are different from the reasons for first-time adoption. Most offices are interested in having a more stable network, with less downtime and better technical support. They also want the additional flexibility of working remotely. First-generation EHR systems may allow files to be viewed from a remote workstation, but they usually don't allow changes to be made.

Migrating data from one electronic record-keeping system to another without losing or corrupting it is no easy task. Nevertheless, legacy transitions tend to cause only a momentary loss of productivity, compared with the prolonged disruption common when a paper-based office goes live on a new system. The users' familiarity with computers in general and with EHR systems in particular makes any serious dislocations unlikely. In addition, workflow processes compatible with an electronic records system are already in place. They may require adjustment, but not overhaul.

Perhaps surprisingly, legacy EHR users tend to be more concerned than new users about patient privacy, given the broader access promised by a new system. But Zandieh and colleagues' most unexpected finding is that resistance to the conversion is even greater among legacy users than among paper-based providers adopting an EHR for the

---

EASING THE TRANSITION 4-2—cont'd

first time. They discovered that champions of second-generation systems often experience stiff resistance from providers and staff who are loyal to the legacy system and apprehensive about learning to use a new one.

Zandieh and colleagues suggest a remedy that's the opposite of what you might expect: They recommend coercion, not cooperation. Collegiality only seems to give reluctant converts a license to whine, fret, and delay—proof, at least, that the original transition from paper to EHR was a success.

Data from Zandieh, S. O., Yoon-Flannery, K., & Kuperman, G. (2008). Challenges to EHR implementation in electronic-versus paper-based office practices. *Journal of General Internal Medicine*, 23(6), 755–761.

Of course, there are no hard-and-fast dividing lines between one type of conversion and another. Conversions take place at a pace ranging from glacial to staggered to full bore, depending on what makes sense for the practice's needs and resources. Some specialty offices chose an unusual but sensible dual-phase deployment in which half of the six orthopedic physicians, and presumably the office staff, went live as the other three providers continued to train on the system. Practices affiliated with large networks may select one or two offices to pilot test a system before introducing it on a larger scale.

The Moguls pursued a modified hybrid approach. Instead of handling existing patients' charts on paper permanently, as in a typical hybrid system, they decided to do so only until the existing patients' files could be added to the EHR system. As soon as a record had been entered electronically, the person's EHR became active, and the paper chart was stored only as an archive.

CRITICAL THINKING EXERCISE 4-3

Do you think the conversion plan designed by The Moguls will work well? What kinds of problems might they be setting themselves up for? What advantages does their staggered rollout plan offer?

SELECTING AN EHR VENDOR AND NETWORK PLATFORM

Hundreds of vendors offer EHR systems for ambulatory (outpatient) care. It's tough not to be swayed by a good sales pitch or wooed by an attentive sales rep. It's important to base the decision on criteria specific to the practice. To do so, providers and staff must take stock of their needs.

Assessing the Practice's Needs

Many of the practice's needs should have been identified during the initial readiness assessment. The physicians at The Moguls identified the following criteria they'd like their EHR system to have:

- They want to choose a company that will be around to provide long-term service, such as software updates and training for new employees.
- They want to choose a system that uses a controlled vocabulary to exchange data, such as lab results and accounting information, with other systems.
- They want to make sure they select an EHR that performs well and meets a wide range of industry specifications; therefore, they want one that is CCHIT certified.
- They want a system that has a variety of customization options. This means that terminology, display menus, templates, and linkages between a patient's history, examination, and diagnoses can all be tailored to the practice's preferences.
- Being a small practice, The Moguls need to keep their investment cost low and their operating costs manageable.

CRITICAL THINKING EXERCISE 4-4

In choosing an EHR system, how might the needs of a dermatology or rheumatology practice differ from those of an orthopedics or obstetric practice? How might the size of the practice influence EHR selection?

Surveying Available Software Applications

Although the amount of EHR **applications software,** or software systems, may seem overwhelming at first, selecting one is really no different from buying a car, an appliance, or any other high-ticket item. A good way to begin is by researching available systems online. The American Academy of Family Physicians (AAFP) publishes an annual EHR user satisfaction survey in which about a dozen of the top software systems are rated according to functionality, ease of use and flexibility, customer service and support, cost, interoperability, and security. You can also talk to users in other offices and read journal articles and news items that outline the experiences other offices have had. Vendors are a good source of information about features, but they have an interest in not disclosing product flaws and limitations.

It's good practice to submit a **request for proposal (RFP)** document after narrowing the list to a handful of vendors. Representatives of each type of user in the practice, such as medical assistants and physicians, should help prepare the RFP. This document gives vendors a detailed picture of the practice setting, environment, needs, expectations, current technologic capabilities and hardware setup, regulatory compliance procedures and concerns, time frame, and budget. In return, each vendor is asked to supply the following specific information to help the practice compare competing vendors and their products side by side:

- **Vendor's software development expertise.** Was the vendor's software developed in-house, or is it just a dealer?
- **Vendor's financial stability.** What evidence can the vendor supply to prove that it will remain in business in order to service the product?
- **References.** The practice should check references from clients for whom the vendor has completed installations. The vendor should also be willing to furnish a list of installations completed in the last year. The practice should speak to some customers who are not on the vendor's list of references.
- **EHR features.** The features section is the meat of the RFP document. It should comprise a series of specific statements about the practice's needs. The RFP for The Moguls, for instance, specified, "Our EHR must accommodate one off-site physician who will connect to the network via a high-speed cable modem" and "Our EHR must interface with our laboratory partner, Medilytica; our preferred imaging center, Adirondack Imaging Partners; and our local hospital, Olympiad Medical Center," and so on.
- **Proposed hardware platform and network architecture.** The vendor's proposal should recommend the appropriate hardware to support the system, taking into account the number of workstations and complexity of the interfaces requested, the practice's budget, and other factors.
- **Customer service.** A lack of emphasis on customer service in a vendor's proposal should be considered a red flag. The proposal should outline a detailed implementation plan, including training and ongoing technical support.
- **Health Insurance Portability and Accountability Act (HIPAA) and coding compliance features.** An EHR should simplify coding and shore up the practice's compliance with HIPAA security and privacy regulations. The vendor's proposal should explain its EHR's compliance features as they apply to the practice's setting. In particular, it should highlight the EHR's security features, such as Smart Card or biometric access.
- **Interoperability functions. Data capture** is much more efficient when the EHR can interface with compatible laboratory systems, accounting databases, and other electronic systems. For most practices this feature weighs heavily in making the final selection.

- **Costs.** All those features can be pricey, so the practice must strike a balance between choosing the features it needs or is likely to need soon and purchasing a program that is more robust than the practice will ever use. The vendor's proposal should provide a detailed cost estimate. This estimate should include an analysis of return on investment (ROI) and a break-even analysis, showing at what point the savings generated by the system makes up for the cost of implementing it. Finally, the proposal should specify the length of the contract required (if a licensed subscription product is chosen) and explain the warranty features (if the software is to be purchased outright).

The staff or EHR selection committee should make its decision as a group, but with the understanding that compromise is essential. There is no such thing as the perfect software, so the practice should select the one that best meets its needs in the most important areas. Let's say your primary reason for EHR adoption is revenue analysis and improvement. In that case, the decision may hinge on coding and accounting features and overall efficiency. If improved health promotion and clinical documentation are the top priorities, then advanced CDS features will be key to the selection.

Contracts with software vendors can be negotiated—don't assume that the vendor's price estimate is the bottom line. The bigger your practice, the more leverage you have in negotiating a better price. You should secure in writing any promises made during phone calls or in person regarding either costs or extras such as training. Even if you have confidence in your rep, he or she may be working for a competitor next week, and casual promises won't mean much to the new guy.

SELECTING A NETWORK PLATFORM

Choosing EHR software also requires selecting a network architecture and appropriate hardware to support the system. These decisions are inseparable from one another. EHR software can be licensed (purchased outright) or accessed by paying a monthly subscription fee to use it (see Table 4-2). In a licensing arrangement, the user purchases the software and installs it on the practice's own server. This is called the **client-server model.** In a subscription arrangement, the user pays a monthly fee to the **application service provider (ASP)** for use of the software application, which it accesses over a secure Internet connection. This eliminates the need for the practice to purchase the software outright, conserving valuable operating funds. It also simplifies the on-site hardware setup (see Table 4-1). This type of provider is also called software as a service (SAAS).

The Moguls chose an EHR under an ASP licensing arrangement. The application (that is, the software) resides at the EHR's central data center, where the data (namely, patient files) are stored. This information is accessed via a secure Internet connection called a **virtual private network (VPN)**, as shown in Figure 4-1. The ASP maintains all server functions, such as installing and updating the software, while the practice sets up and maintains the hardware and network on its end.

Table 4-2 *Application Service Provider (ASP) Networks vs. Client-Server Applications (CSA)*

	Costs	
Attribute	**ASP**	**CSA**
Initial investment	Hardware, local networking systems, and connectivity must be purchased and the software licensing fee paid. A hub computer is generally used to link examination-room workstations, other accessory workstations, and printers.	A more robust server and compatible hardware must be purchased up front, requiring a large cash outlay. This arrangement is more appropriate for large practices.
Operating costs	Monthly subscription fees depend on the number of workstations and typically include software updates, IT support, and server maintenance.	New software or updates will have to be purchased as technology improves and EHR standards evolve. In addition, administration costs are borne by the practice rather than included in the subscription fee.

Table 4-2 *Application Service Provider (ASP) Networks vs. Client-Server Applications (CSA)—cont'd*

Attribute	ASP	CSA
		Costs
Implementation and training fees	To help the client get the system and its users up and running, ASPs often charge an implementation and training fee, plus travel expenses, based on the number of providers in the practice. This fee also covers the cost of customizing the software to suit the needs of the practice.	These costs are highly variable; check with the software vendor before signing a contract.
Access	Ability to access the EHR from any location with an Internet connection, including home offices, hospitals, and even hotel rooms when the providers are attending conferences.	Remote access can be achieved only with remote-access tools such as "Go to my PC" and "PC Anywhere."
Flexibility	ASPs often require users to sign a contract agreeing to purchase at least a year's worth of service. After that time the contract can usually be terminated, but plans will have to be made to migrate patients' records securely to a dedicated server or to another ASP.	Because purchasing software requires a large initial investment, the practice has little recourse if the system does not suit its needs. However, a client-server arrangement can accommodate a broader selection of administrator options.
Privacy and security	User authentication measures (see Chapter 3) are used to verify that a user has legitimate access to the system. Data are backed up by secure, redundant T1 lines with high-speed Internet connections. The data are sent through a VPN that securely encrypts the data during transmission.	Because an internal server is used, data are not transmitted over an Internet connection, and encryption technology is not needed; thus CSAs are more secure than ASPs.
Ownership of patient data	The ASP service agreement must specify that the practice owns patient data because the data are stored on the ASP's server.	The practice owns the patient data, and no special agreement or contract is needed.
Start-up time	Depends on the number of providers and staff in the practice and how much training they require, but generally takes about 60 days from software purchase to system start-up.	Depends on the hardware already in place, the server selected, the size of the practice, and other factors. Generally the start-up time is longer than for ASPs.
Reliability	Depends on the reliability of the Internet connection and the ability of the on-site hardware to handle the system. In general, if the hardware and server are compatible, reliability is excellent with a high-speed DSL line.	Depends on the stability of the internal server and its associated hardware; does not depend on having a reliable Internet connection.

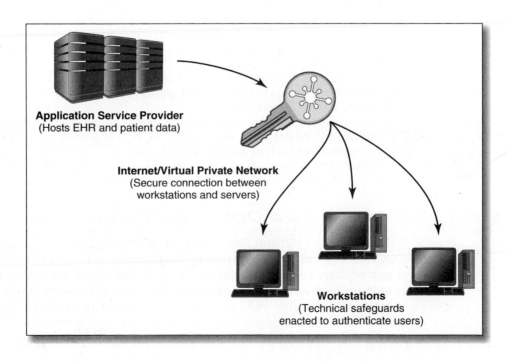

Figure 4-1
Diagram of an application service provider network.

Application Service Provider
(Hosts EHR and patient data)

Internet/Virtual Private Network
(Secure connection between workstations and servers)

Workstations
(Technical safeguards enacted to authenticate users)

The main workstation at The Moguls is the office manager's PC, located in the reception area. Accessory workstations were set up for the nurse practitioner and the three on-site physicians, using tablet PCs wirelessly connected to printers. The medical assistants work with wireless-equipped laptops. The remote physician accesses the EHR from his laptop computer, using a cable modem to connect to the Internet. The Moguls expect to **go live** within 8 weeks of signing a contract with the software vendor.

REDESIGNING WORKFLOW

It's important to perceive EHR adoption not just as the launch of some fancy new technology but as a wholesale shift in the way the office conducts its business. Although the technology must be chosen to suit the user's environment and should not be imposed on it, a significant redesign of staff and clinician **workflow** is inevitable. A workflow is a set of related tasks needed to complete a step in a business process. Various resources are needed to complete such tasks, including people, information, documents (such as the templates in an EHR system), and tools (such as computers).

The EHR vendor should be able to offer sound workflow recommendations. The practice should address workflow redesign in advance, as part of the preimplementation planning process, for every routine function the office performs. The EHR simplifies many workflow processes, such as patient callbacks. In an electronic practice, the provider can access the patient's chart with a couple of mouse clicks rather than wait for a chart-pull.

Box 4-1 lists workflow processes that typically require redesign. However, overhauling the office workflow is not a tidy process. Until the staff has some real-life experience using the software, it's difficult to understand how to integrate it effectively into office processes. The keys to success are flexibility, communication about what's working and what's not, and a willingness to make continual readjustments on the fly.

BOX 4-1
Office Procedures Requiring Workflow Redesign

- Prescription ordering
- Telephone messaging
- Receipt, documentation, and review of lab results
- Recording of vital signs
- Maintenance of to-do lists
- Review of clinical notes
- Patient appointment scheduling, cancellations, no-shows, and waiting lists
- Patient check-in and rooming
- Patient encounters (decide whether and how a computer will be used during visits)
- Patient notification of lab results, imaging results, and care reminders
- Physician on-call scheduling
- Documentation of new-patient information, including insurance information
- Orders and referrals
- Authorizations and medical records requests
- HIPAA compliance

Adjusting to Point-of-Care Documentation

Perhaps the most difficult new workflow for some clinicians to adapt to is point-of-care (POC) documentation, which means that documentation is done by the provider during or immediately after the patient encounter. Paper offices use a variety of documentation techniques, such as dictation and transcription, but documentation is generally completed after the patient's visit. POC documentation may increase the burden on providers, who used to be able to delegate many documentation activities. However, once mastered, practitioners may appreciate the reduction in their after-hours paperwork.

CRITICAL THINKING EXERCISE 4-5

Which documentation activities are delegated in a paper-based office? How, specifically, might this workflow be redesigned for EHR implementation in your office or in a typical general practitioner's office?

Setting Up Billing Cycle Documentation

Standardized diagnosis and procedure codes are transmitted to the practice's billing system or to an external accounting vendor. The codes must be correct or reimbursement will be affected and the practice may be subject to accusations of fraud and abuse. This coding is part of the documentation process. Documentation and workflow in the EHR must be arranged to avoid constructing systems that are inadvertently fraudulent. This can happen, for instance, if the automatic sign-off function is improperly used to indicate that a provider has reviewed a batch of documents rather than verifying them one at a time. The provider's electronic signature may be considered fraudulent because the entire batch would bear the same time and date—a physical impossibility. This can also happen when a physician signs electronically for services provided by a nurse practitioner or medical assistant, thus increasing the claims value of the service provided.

When a practice converts to an EHR, it must identify potential glitches in claims processing and reimbursement or be prepared to sort out such problems once they're discovered. The practice management capabilities of an EHR system are extremely useful in performing ongoing financial analysis and billing management functions. The American Health Information Management Association (AHIMA) makes the following recommendations for practices that are going digital:

- Determine which diagnosis and procedure codes are used most frequently, and ensure that quality measures are tied to them in the EHR.
- Take advantage of the system's auditing and reporting capabilities to make sure documentation is thorough, accurate, and consistent; put in place plans for improvement when it's not.
- Pay particular attention to the accuracy and completeness of diagnosis and procedure codes, which must be kept up to date. AHIMA recommends using a health information management (HIM) professional to make sure codes are current and to test billing system function. Such expert advice is certainly advisable and may be cost effective in the long term. However, the cost of hiring such professionals may be steep and adds to the expense of migrating from paper to an EHR.
- Set standards, in accordance with all applicable laws and regulations, for what constitutes a complete and compliant record and for how long it should take to complete adequate documentation. Although much documentation is done at the point of care, progress notes and other entries may need to be reviewed for clinical accuracy (for example, a nurse practitioner's documentation may be verified by a physician) or to ensure that coding is correct.
- Design the EHR to avoid shortcuts that leave the practice vulnerable to accusations of fraud or malpractice. Pressed for time, providers may copy and paste clinical notes from a previous visit into the current progress note or copy and paste notes from one patient's record into the record of a patient with a similar presentation. These practices are called **cloning** or "carrying forward," and they're an invitation to accusations of sloppy patient care and fraudulent claims submission because they give a static account of clinical findings and may trigger billing for treatment not rendered.
- Set up workflow processes for both regularly scheduled and random auditing. The audits should verify, at a minimum, the following:
  - Data capture and documentation are accurate.
  - Procedures performed or services rendered are consistent with the conditions diagnosed and treatment or services billed.

- Progress notes show no evidence of cloning.
- Electronic signatures and auto-authentication functions are being used appropriately.
- Prescribing activities are transparent and well documented.

AHIMA has released a position statement on billing cycle documentation in the EHR, available online to AHIMA members.

COLLECTING DATA

Most of the data initially entered into the EHR come from the paper chart. However, to offer the best possible healthcare and to protect the practice legally, it's important to gather patient data from all available sources, within reason. Information may be available from computer networks that belong to an affiliated hospital. For example, the hospital's lab, pharmacy, or billing department may have electronic records on file. Some departments may have hard-copy forms that can be scanned or keyed into the newly created EHR. The Moguls often sent patients to a nearby imaging center for computed tomography (CT) scans and magnetic resonance imaging (MRI), and those data were added to the practice's own records.

ENTERING DATA

The need to key data from paper charts into the new EHR is one of the biggest deterrents to adopting an EHR system. Going digital essentially makes every patient a new patient until his or her record has been keyed into the system. As discussed in Chapter 1, information from paper charts may be entered into the EHR in one of four ways:

1. Data input from compatible, interfaced systems
2. Transcription using voice recognition technology or dictation
3. Scanning of typed or handwritten documents
4. Direct keying or re-keying (typing)

Under-documentation and Over-documentation

Transferring extensive documentation from paper charts to the EHR is time consuming, and each method has specific drawbacks, such as the potential for dictation errors and the impossibility of scanning illegible handwriting. To streamline the data entry process, some practices enter information selectively. Doing so, however, requires the clinical judgment of a physician, nurse practitioner, or other person with medical training.

In addition, when too little information is entered, the skimpy EHR tends to generate drug interaction alerts and health promotion reminders more often. If these red flags become too numerous, they can be like horseflies—absently batted away and then forgotten until they come back to bite you. Over-documentation, on the other hand, carries risks as well. Excessive detail may indicate a higher level of care than that actually delivered, leaving the provider vulnerable to charges of fraud and abuse.

In selectively transferring information from paper charts to EHR systems, clinicians should prioritize the types of information to be entered. At The Moguls, all medication lists, allergy information, and test results less than 3 years old, for example, were given a higher priority than notations regarding episodic illnesses (colds and flu, for instance) and certain other types of information. Medication lists more than 3 years old were deemed low priority. This allowed the practice to begin populating established patients' electronic files with the most critical information first.

Structured and Unstructured Data Entry

Unlike paper charts, EHR systems rely on a **controlled vocabulary** for efficient **structured data entry.** Structured data entry is a useful way of recording straightforward clinical findings quickly, but the terminology may be inadequately individualized to capture the nuances of complex or unusual clinical presentations. In such situations, **unstructured data entry** allows the provider to describe the patient's history and condition freely and fully. In fact, to comply with evaluation and management (E/M) guidelines for establishing medical necessity, unstructured data entry is mandatory.

Unstructured data entry provides a thorough and accurate description of the patient's clinical presentation, helps flesh out the patient's yes or no answers to questions about history and review of systems, and describes abnormal findings on physical examination. Finally, it allows the provider to give an overall clinical impression and explain the rationale for recommending or prescribing a given treatment. Dictation templates, a type of EHR template that suggests points to cover without supplying full sentences, lie somewhere between structured and unstructured data entry. SimChart for the Medical Office (SCMO) will offer students a full range of experience using both structured and unstructured data entry options throughout the system.

EHR DISCUSSION 4-1:   TEMPLATES

Use the Simulation Playground and select and review the Missed Appointment template from the Letters section of the Correspondence info panel. Next, select the Blank Letter template. After reviewing, consider the advantages and disadvantages of using templates in the medical office.

Electronic Misfiling

A common documentation problem, both during the EHR transition and afterward, is electronic misfiling. Electronic misfiling is the digital equivalent of physically misfiling a document—in other words, information is recorded in the wrong part of the chart. To prevent this problem, larger EHR systems sometimes mark documents with bar codes that automatically direct them to the right part of the EHR.

Interfacing

Using a controlled vocabulary, most EHR software systems can interface with at least some other systems, such as a hospital or laboratory system. When this interface is seamless, reports from one system automatically populate templates in another. They will also populate applicable letter templates, such as the cholesterol results letter template.

However, ensuring the compatibility of the EHR system's interfaces requires advanced technical knowledge. Moreover, incompatibilities are still common. Consequently, when making referrals and selecting vendors (such as imaging centers and labs), an EHR-equipped practice may be inclined to use or recommend those that offer compatible systems.

SCHEDULING TRAINING

Before training begins, the staff should agree on customization options and set them. If screen views, navigation options, and templates are altered later, users will have to relearn how to use them. The EHR vendor can guide the selection and modification of customized features. Customization can be a time-consuming process, taking perhaps several weeks for a practice to review the existing system and make appropriate changes or additions.

Training may seem like a straightforward concept, but it means different things to different EHR users depending on their level of computer experience. Those who have never used a computer may need instruction on how to use a mouse, resize screens, navigate using a web browser and search engine, click on links, copy and paste, drag and drop, use screen icons, and select from drop-down menus. But even those who are computer savvy may not have used a tablet PC before. Some users may find it worth the time to take a basic keyboarding (typing) course.

administrators, the practice has contracted with a local company called Computer Commandos to provide as-needed support for complex issues.

IMPLEMENTING THE TRANSITION

Heavy doses of patience and humor will be required as the implementation phase begins. The launch and rollout, whether it's a staggered approach or all at once, should be thought of almost as a test phase. As such, flexibility is critical. Finger pointing and blame should be replaced with a "What can we learn from this?" attitude. If adequate planning has been done and contingency plans have been made, few problems will be serious enough to bring the office to a standstill.

Readiness to launch the implementation phase depends on the installation of technologic resources, the completion of staff training, the existence of funding to carry the practice through the transition period, and the availability of staff and clinicians. In addition, during the launch and for some time afterward, depending on the clinic's size, previous technologic abilities, and needs, IT support must be available for troubleshooting. This support may take the form of an on-site vendor representative, online and telephone support, or one or more staff members who have been trained to anticipate and resolve technical problems.

As the EHR is put into use, the plan for its implementation is tested. Its limitations quickly become apparent. The process of soliciting input from all staff members and providers can be useful once again in bringing to light any bottlenecks, security gaps, compliance issues, or other problems; analyzing their causes; and customizing the EHR to work around or accommodate them.

MEASURING RESULTS AND CONDUCTING ONGOING EVALUATIONS

The use of EHR systems has been associated with improved safety and patient care, better financial performance, higher provider satisfaction, and more efficient communication. Improved financial performance is relatively easy to measure after implementation because most paper-based practices track expenses and income, providing a basis for comparison when the EHR is implemented. Practices generally have lower costs for records storage, fewer denied insurance claims, shorter reimbursement cycles, decreased transcription costs, and perhaps lower premiums for malpractice insurance because many insurance companies now offer incentives for going digital. An EHR helps providers qualify for certain quality improvement incentives because the system makes outcomes easy to track.

Improvement in quality of patient care is usually measured in terms of how well care conforms to nationally recognized standards for various conditions, such as the treatment of diabetes and heart disease. Insurance companies and Medicare offer financial incentives to providers who adhere to these standards. This system is known as *pay for performance*.

Medical practices can use the CDS tools in their EHR to track quality measures not necessarily linked to reimbursement, such as the percentage of eligible patients in the practice who have received a flu vaccination. However, a pre- and postimplementation comparison of quality of patient care, effectiveness of communication, efficiency, and other quality attributes can be tricky. After all, most paper-based practices have no means of accurately measuring performance in these areas. And if no preimplementation data exist, there is no basis for comparison after implementation.

As soon as an EHR goes live, though, the system begins to generate baseline data that will allow later comparisons and show trends over time. The Moguls, for instance, want to improve patient communication. They decide to begin by tracking the percentage of patients who receive follow-up letters summarizing their visit. Thirty days after the rollout, a report shows that only 40% of patients received such letters during the first month the EHR was in place. The Moguls have set a goal of doubling that percentage within 1 year. A year from now they can run the numbers again to see whether they've accomplished their goal.

The attributes that can be measured with an EHR are nearly unlimited. EHR systems can show the number of referrals given, hospital admissions made, and prescriptions written. They can determine which provider sees the most patients. They can indicate which examination rooms are underused and how many no-shows the practice tends to have before holiday weekends. In fact, when staff members and providers discover just how versatile an EHR system is, most of them reach the same conclusion: *We could never go back to paper.*

CHAPTER SUMMARY

- A successful transition from paper charts to an EHR system requires consideration of the practice's expectations, organizational culture, budget, and existing resources. During the preimplementation process, the practice should assess its needs and expectations, set a budget, and outline a time frame from initial research to the go-live date. On the go-live date the practice may switch entirely to an EHR system, begin an intermittent transition, or enter only new patients into the EHR (called a *hybrid approach*). Many variations of these options are possible, depending on the practice's needs.
- The meaningful use incentive program is available to eligible providers who meet the required core and menu objectives established by CMS.
- A conversion plan generally includes setting up a focus group of office staff, researching other practice transitions, deciding whether the office will be hybrid or full EHR, and designing a transfer of records approach.
- Research into EHR software usually requires preparation of an RFP document. This is a formal request for each vendor to supply detailed information about its reliability and financial stability, the features and functionality of its product, its proposed preimplementation plan, and estimated costs.
- When a practice adopts an EHR system, nearly every workflow process in the office must be redesigned. New workflow processes should be outlined and practiced during the preimplementation phase and adjusted after the EHR goes live.
- Some data entered into the new EHR may need to be collected from external sources such as hospitals. The need to transfer data from paper charts to the EHR's electronic files is one of the chief barriers to implementing an EHR system in the medical practice. Data can be entered via interfaced systems, transcription, scanning, or typing.
- Under-documentation, over-documentation, and electronic misfiling are common problems when information is transferred from paper charts to an EHR system.
- Training to use an EHR system may range from learning to use a mouse and web browser to learning to apply the EHR's advanced functions.
- Both the staff and the clinician, if possible, should introduce patients to the new EHR system by following the three C's recommended by CMS: connect, collaborate, and close.
- Before an EHR system is launched, the practice must make contingency plans to protect patients' data.
- Readiness to implement the EHR depends on having the necessary technologic resources in place, completing staff training, and arranging for funding to carry the practice through a period of reduced productivity.
- Once an EHR has been launched, results can be gauged both in financial terms and in terms of quality of care delivered.

CHAPTER REVIEW ACTIVITIES

Key Terms Review

Match the term in column A to the definition in column B.

1. Records management
2. Organizational culture
3. Legacy EHR
4. Hybrid
5. Virtual private network (VPN)
6. Workflow
7. Unstructured data entry
8. Template
9. Go live
10. Cloning
11. Controlled vocabulary
12. Client-server model

a. A medical practice in which health records are stored using some combination of paper and electronic media

b. Free-text keying of data directly into the electronic record

c. To leave the practice mode and become operational

d. The systematic control of patient records, from creation through maintenance and storage

e. A platform in which a powerful central computer serves a network of connected PCs or other workstations

f. A pathway that allows encrypted data to travel securely through an Internet connection to its destination, where it is unencrypted

g. Copying and pasting information from a previous entry in the patient's record or from another patient's record

h. The shared set of values, beliefs, and assumptions that governs behavior and decision making within a healthcare practice

i. A standardized list of preferred terms and corresponding codes for medical diagnoses, findings, procedures, services, and treatments

j. Predefined, customizable forms that speed structured data collection

k. A set of related tasks necessary to complete a step in a business process

l. An existing, functional EHR system scheduled to be replaced with a newer software application

True/False

Indicate whether the statement is true or false.

1. _____ To simplify the preimplementation process, only key decision makers and a staff representative should be involved.

2. _____ A legacy EHR is a failed EHR system left behind when the staff gives up on learning how to use it.

3. _____ Software vendors should be the practice's only source of information about the product because no one knows the application better.

4. _____ HIPAA compliance and security features should be considered in choosing an EHR system.

5. _____ Client-server platforms are generally more expensive to start up than ASP licensing arrangements.

6. _____ Workflow redesign will not be addressed until the EHR system goes live.

7. _____ Fraud can occur if an EHR is not properly designed to accommodate the practice's financial documentation.

8. _____ Audits should be conducted both randomly and at regular intervals under security plans.

9. _____ Over-documentation can leave a provider vulnerable to charges of fraud and abuse.

10. _____ Electronic misfiling is the digital equivalent of physically misfiling a document.

11. _____ Interfacing has made incompatible systems a thing of the past because all systems are now interoperable.

12. _____ The best approach to training is a sink-or-swim attitude because users learn best when they have to figure things out for themselves.

13. _____ Patients are unlikely to notice the conversion from paper to an EHR.

14. _____ Backing up data in the patient's EHR is mandated by HIPAA.

15. _____ Providers starting the meaningful use program in 2014 will not have to meet the stage 1 requirements before moving on to stage 2.

Workplace Applications

Using the knowledge you obtained from the chapter, provide narrative answers to the following cases.

1. How well does the organizational culture in your office support the use of technology? What is the medical assistant's role in supporting new technology in the medical office? What specific steps could you take to become a stronger advocate for healthcare technology in general and for EHR use in particular?

2. Why should medical assistants be part of the EHR selection committee and the preimplementation team? What specific contributions can they make? Describe how you might take a leadership role in the EHR transition process.

3. Your office is converting to EHR. You are in charge of the conversion process. Use the Conversion Plan posted to Evolve Resources to complete a Conversion Plan.

4. Select and explain three Core objectives and three Menu objectives required under the stage 2 meaningful use incentive program.

5. Use the Internet to research five EHR vendors. Complete the EHR Vendor Research table located in Evolve Student Resources to rate each system.

6. Develop a transition letter that will go out to Dr. Walden and Martin's patients that will inform their patients of EHR implementation. Use the Blank Letter Template in the SCMO Form Repository.

BIBLIOGRAPHY

AHIMA Work Group on Electronic Health Records Management. (2004). The strategic importance of electronic health records management: Checklist for transition to the EHR. *Journal of American Health Information Management Association*, 75(9), 80C–80E.

AHIMA. (2008). Quality data and documentation for EHRs in physician practice. *Journal of American Health Information Management Association*, 79(8), 43–48.

Baron, R. J., Fabens, E. L., & Schiffman, M., et al. (2005). Electronic health records: Just around the corner? Or over the cliff? *Annals of Internal Medicine*, 143(3), 222–226.

Bates, D. W. (2006). The road to implementation of the electronic health record. *Baylor University Medical Center Proceedings* (Vol. 19, 4, pp. 311–312). Available at: http://www.baylorhealth.edu/Documents/BUMC%20Proceedings/2006%20Vol%2019/No.%204/19_4_Bates.pdf. Accessed 24.03.08.

Denny, S. (2008). Queuing up for quality: Boosting quality with electronic work queues. *Journal of American Health Information Management Association*, 79(1), 32–36.

DesRoches, C. M, Campbell, E. G, Rao, S.R, et al. (2008). Electronic health records in ambulatory care—A national survey of doctors. *The New England Journal of Medicine*, 359, 50–60.

Dimick, C. (2008). Documentation bad habits: Shortcuts in electronic records pose risk. *Journal of American Health Information Management Association*, 79(6), 40–43.

Fullerton, C., Aponte, P., Hopkins, R. III, et al. (2006). Lessons learned from pilot site implementation of an ambulatory electronic health record. *Baylor University Medical Center Proceedings* October 2006; 19(4): 303–310.

Grzybowski, D. (2008). Storage solution: A plan for paper in the transition to electronic document management. *Journal of American Health Information Management Association*, 79(5), 44–47. Available at http://library.ahima.org/xpedio/groups/public/documents/ahima/bok1_038089.hcsp?dDocName =bok1_038089. Accessed 11.06.11.

Hsu, J. (2008). *Why hasn't EHR been adopted faster?* Gerson Lehman Group: November 26, Available at: www.glgroup.com/News/Why-hasnt-EHR-been-adopted-faster-29330.html. Accessed 03.01.09.

Menachemi, N., Ettel, D. L., Brooks, R. G., et al. (2006). Charting the use of electronic health records and other information technologies among child health providers. *BMC Pediatrics*, 6(21). Available at: www. pubmedcentral.nih.gov/articlerender.fcgi?tool=pubmed&;pubmedid=16869972. Accessed 24.03.14.

Morrison, D. P. (2006). Lead—don't manage—EHR adoption: allowing multiple work processes leads to unnecessary inefficiencies. *Behavioral Healthcare* 26(1), 36-37. Available at www.behavioral.net/ME2/d irmod.asp?nm=Archives&;type=Publishing&mod=Publications%3A%3AArticle&mid=64D490AC6A7 D4FE1AEB453627F1A4A32&tier=4&id=36D1D845F35C42F7A4840BB2A99C2C9D. Accessed 11.06.11.

Terry, A. L., Thorpe, C. F., Giles, G., et al. (2008). Implementing electronic health records: Key factors in primary care. *Canadian Family Doctor Medecin de Famille Canadien*, 54(5), 730–736. Available at: www. pubmedcentral.nih.gov/articlerender.fcgi?tool=pubmed&;pubmedid=18474707. Accessed 04.01.09.

chapter 5

Administrative Use of the Electronic Health Record

Chapter Outline

Commission on Accreditation of Allied Health Education Programs (CAAHEP) Competencies

1. Explain general office policies.
2. Demonstrate telephone techniques.
3. Document patient care.
4. Compose professional/business letters.
5. Discuss the pros and cons of various types of appointment management systems.
6. Describe scheduling guidelines.
7. Recognize office policies and protocols for handling appointments.
8. Identify systems for organizing medical records.
9. Discuss principles of using the electronic medical record (EMR).
10. Manage the appointment schedule, using established priorities.
11. Execute data management using electronic health records (EHR) such as the EMR.

Chapter Objectives

1. Explain the importance and typical duties of the front office assistant.
2. Discuss the necessity of respectful communication among providers, staff, and patients when answering the telephone, sending email, messaging, faxing, and scheduling appointments.
3. Create a telephone message in the SimChart for the Medical Office (SCMO).
4. Explain why a provider might send a letter to a healthcare provider or patient, and learn how to create one in an EHR.

5. Generate patient correspondence in SCMO.
6. Outline the procedure for the management of EHRs, including eliminating duplicate charts, the proper way of purging closed patient records, and the importance of backing up the EHR.
7. Create and manage patient appointments in the calendar.
8. Discuss the role of the front office in maintaining the waiting room.

Key Terms

double-booking   Giving two or more patients the same appointment slot with the same provider.

encryption technology   A system that keeps data secure by converting it to an unreadable code during transmission and then unencrypting the information when it reaches the recipient.

fax machine   A device capable of encoding documents and sending them over a telephone line; a secure fax sends fax transmissions via secure email, eliminating many of a fax's security risks.

no-show   A patient who makes an appointment and neither shows up nor calls to cancel; the term also refers to the appointment itself (a "no-show appointment").

patient flow   The efficient movement of patients through the medical office as a product of accurately estimated patient volume, a consistent provider pace, and efficient scheduling practices; the term generally refers to the overall flow of patients but can refer to the path of an individual patient.

purging   The process of separating inactive patient health records from active ones.

secure email   An email system capable of transmitting an encrypted message and storing it in a coded format until it is retrieved by the recipient via a secure web link.

show rate   The percentage of patients in a practice who arrive for appointments as scheduled or call in advance to cancel or reschedule.

telephone etiquette   A polite, helpful response and respectful manner toward callers that shows patients they are cared for and valued.

views   Different ways of displaying the same or similar information on a computer screen, usually with an increasing or decreasing level of detail (for example, looking at an electronic calendar in daily, weekly, and monthly views).

ROLE OF THE FRONT OFFICE ASSISTANT

Every pharmaceutical rep knows that the real person to win over in a medical practice is not the physician, but the front office assistant. After all, if the rep can't get past the reception window, he or she won't have a chance to impress the physician with that spiel on beta blockers.

But front office assistants are more than just people who guard the moat. They play a complex, important role, and they must be well trained and versatile to do so. Most important, they must have a great attitude toward patients, providers, and staff. We have all been patients at a medical office where the staff members treat patients like unwelcome interruptions rather than valued healthcare customers. Perhaps some of us have worked in an environment where staff members pass the time by making fun of patients behind their backs rather than by figuring out ways to make an often distressing experience more pleasant. Fortunately, such offices are rare. However, it takes just one person with a poor attitude and a strong personality to taint the atmosphere for everyone else. Patients pick up on such attitudes, and many of these dissatisfied customers, so to speak, don't return.

CRITICAL THINKING EXERCISE 5-1

What are the consequences for a practice if patients don't return because of what might be called customer service issues? In your answer, consider the impact on staff, providers, patient care, and practice revenue.

The front office is usually where patients get their first impression of the medical office. Staff members must be ready to help with anything the physician asks of them, within the bounds of ethics, law, and common sense. Primary front office duties usually include:
- Greeting patients on the phone and in person
- Creating and managing an EHR for each patient
- Generating patient letters and other correspondence
- Maintaining the office schedule.
- Providing patients with and updating registration forms.

COMMUNICATION IN THE MEDICAL OFFICE

Good communication among providers, patients, and staff improves patients' confidence in their care and increases their satisfaction with the medical practice. It also makes healthcare personnel feel better about their jobs, which has been shown to lower staff and clinician turnover. But good communication does more than just give everyone the warm fuzzies. Studies have proven it also prevents many medical errors, thus improving care and reducing the incidence of malpractice lawsuits. But here's the astonishing part: Good communication is so important, it actually reduces the likelihood a patient will bring a lawsuit even when a medical error is made.

The explanation for this phenomenon is simple—patients or family members who file lawsuits tend to be upset not so much that a mistake was made but that no one ever apologized for the error and the harm it caused. This seems intuitively true for other kinds of mistakes—we're a lot more miffed about an undercooked steak if the waiter says "It wasn't my fault" than if he simply says he's sorry. Likewise, as Levinson and colleagues discovered in their classic 1997 study of this topic, it's neither the error nor the poor communication alone, but the toxic combination of the two that triggers malpractice suits.

Although such studies have focused primarily on physician-patient encounters, staff interaction is important in making patients feel valued and comfortable. Levinson and colleagues found that patients appreciate being informed, for example, of what to expect. Front office assistants can play a key role in orienting patients during their visits.

The Health Insurance Portability and Accountability Act (HIPAA) Privacy Rule allows medical practices and other covered entities to disclose healthcare information via email, fax, or phone without specific patient authorization, provided reasonable care is taken to avoid inappropriate disclosure or use of protected health information (PHI). If you can't tell whether the last digit of a handwritten fax number is a "7" or a "2," for instance, a reasonable safeguard might be to call the patient to verify the number before sending the fax.

Communication within the medical office and between patients and healthcare professionals is continually evolving. Some medical offices now offer patient portals as a way of giving patients the option of viewing open slots on the schedule and making their own appointments online rather than having to call and ask which dates and times are available.

In the following sections we'll explore some specific means of communicating in today's medical office setting.

CRITICAL THINKING EXERCISE 5-2

We've given an example of a reasonable safeguard you might take when sending PHI by fax. Can you think of safeguards you might need to take when calling a patient to let her know the results of a pregnancy test? What precautions might be necessary when emailing instructions to a home care nurse assigned to visit an oncology patient in your practice?

Patient Correspondence

A variety of types of correspondence can be created within the EHR, including physician referral letters, patient letters, and patient instructions. Providers may want to write a letter to a patient (e.g., to inform of test results or to summarize a plan of care), or they may want to send a letter about a patient (for instance, to provide a consultation report).

Letters in EHR systems can be prepared from standard letter templates, preconstructed documents that address specific topics but can be customized for individual recipients. Templates keep providers and assistants from having to compose an original letter every time they send correspondence on a topic such as cholesterol results and medical record requests.

Many EHR systems also have functionality that enables the staff to create their own letters from the clinical documentation in the chart using macros, embedded instruction codes that automatically gather information from the patient's demographics, case information, encounter information, orders, provider's history and examination notes, nursing documentation, prescribed medications, future appointments, referral orders to specialists, and aftercare instructions. For example, let's say you work for a specialist who treats burn patients, and you write letters to the referring physicians to update them about a patient's progress. By entering the term [body_surface_area] into a letter template, the EHR will automatically use the patient's height and weight to calculate the patient's body surface area and enter it into the letter.

Physician Referral

Often a particular physician lacks the expertise or proper credentials to treat a patient with a specific condition. The provider will send the patient to a board-certified physician for specialized treatment, testing, or consultation. This is called a referral.

The referring physician will complete a referral form to give the specialist a clear picture of the patient's general health, health history, and the condition for which the patient is seeking care. Once the specialist has seen the patient, he or she will contact the referring physician by phone or letter to outline the treatment plan. Trends and Applications 5-1 describes some benefits of copying referral letters and similar correspondence to patients.

TRENDS AND APPLICATIONS 5-1

The Copy Letter: Should We Follow the Brits' Lead?

In 2005 the United Kingdom's National Health Service (NHS) began implementing a recommendation that patients receive copies of referrals sent to their general practitioners (GPs) after hospital consultations. Should physicians in the United States follow the United Kingdom's lead and voluntarily send referral copies to patients?

Baxter and colleagues identified four primary reasons that physicians are uncomfortable copying communication to patients. First, they worry such communication might make patients anxious about their condition. Second, they believe patients may have difficulty understanding medical terminology and don't wish to translate the information. Third, they worry that misdirected communication might violate the patient's privacy rights. Fourth, providers cite the additional workload and associated copying costs.

The first concern has not been borne out by research. Krishna and Damato interviewed patients with ocular (eye) cancer who were referred to super-specialized cancer physicians called *ocular oncologists*. The purpose of the study was to see how patients with a particularly stressful diagnosis would react to being given the additional information contained in the referral sent by the ocular oncologist to their GPs and to the referring ophthalmologist. Rather than finding the referral stressful, the patients remarked that the explanations of their condition helped them accept it. Most used the letter as a jumping off point to discuss the diagnosis with their family and friends. In fact, the researchers found that 97% of patients appreciated receiving copies of the letters.

In addition, patients have shown little difference in comprehension of letters written in medical jargon compared with those written in lay language. Among the cancer patients interviewed by Krishna and Damato, only 17% said they'd like to have the medical terms explained to them.

TRENDS AND APPLICATIONS 5-1—cont'd

As to the other concerns mentioned in the study by Baxter and colleagues, HIPAA allows practitioners to communicate with patients by mail unless they specify otherwise. And finally, studies have shown that copies impose little additional burden on medical assistants and office budgets.

But why go to the extra trouble at all? Well, there are several reasons for sending copies to patients. Let's take a quick inventory:

- Promotes respect and trust between patient and provider
- Better informs patients about why they are being referred, which improves follow-up and compliance with the specialist's recommendations
- Allows patients to become more involved in their healthcare and to take responsibility for making informed choices
- Improves documentation both for the provider who copies the referrals to patients and for the specialist physician who sends patients a copy of the plan of care he or she shares with the patient's GP
- Encourages accuracy because patients have an opportunity to review the practitioner's notes, in effect, and thus correct any misinformation, such as dates of surgery and medication dosages
- Promotes a two-way exchange of information rather than an authoritative, top-down communication process
- Gives the provider an additional chance to communicate information about health promotion and healthy living

Remember, it's a snap to craft communication in an EHR because you can design templates that populate automatically with information from the patient's chart. Of course, providers in the United States aren't required to share their correspondence with patients. But as discussed in Chapter 4, meaningful use stage 2 requirements do require physicians to provide visit summaries, which can be helpful to improving the communication process as well.

A referral is different from a consultation. A consultation, according to the Centers for Medicare & Medicaid Services (CMS), occurs when a physician requests advice or an opinion from another physician or other qualified practitioner regarding the evaluation or management of a specific problem. After a referral, treatment of the condition for which the patient was referred is transferred to the specialist physician. (Occasionally one specialist refers a patient to another specialist in a different or more highly specialized field. For example, a gynecologist might refer a patient to a gynecologic oncologist for treatment of ovarian cancer.)

EHR EXERCISE 5-1:   CREATE A PATIENT REFERRAL

*Complete the following exercise in the EHR exercise environment of SCMO.

Noemi Rodriguez (11/04/1971) is being referred to a cardiologist to perform an echocardiogram 99307 for mitral valve prolapse (MVP) ICD-10-CM I34.1. According to past office notes, the patient has experienced palpitations over the past 2 months. There have been no previous treatments for the MVP. Noemi has no known allergies and takes only a multivitamin daily. The echocardiogram will be performed at Cardiology Associates, located at 445 Heart Valve Way, Anytown, AL 12345. This procedure will take one visit and will be done as an outpatient procedure. Dr. Walden is the referring provider. The NPI number is 8788012880 and the authorization number is NNP3234. It expires 30 days from today. Use the Referral located in Form Repository to complete this activity. Once complete, save the document. You can access this saved form anytime by using the Patient Dashboard (see Chapter 2).

Patient Letter

Physicians send letters to patients for many reasons. For example, if the medical assistant is unable to reach the patient by phone, the patient may be contacted by letter. New patients are often sent a welcome letter, which outlines the office's general policies and procedures for the new patients. Appointment reminders and discharge letters are also examples of patient correspondence.

Occasionally letters are used to address unpleasant matters that must be put in writing for the legal protection of the practice. A request for payment of a delinquent balance is an example. A less common situation occurs when patients must be formally notified that they are being dismissed from the practice (usually because they continually miss appointments and disregard providers' treatment plans).

EHR EXERCISES 5-2:   PATIENT LETTER

*Complete the following exercise in the EHR exercises environment of SCMO.

It is office policy to send all new patients a new patient welcome letter. Susannah Ling (01/02/1973) has recently joined Walden-Martin Family Medical Clinic. Prepare a new patient welcome letter for Susannah Ling.

1. Click on the Correspondence icon.

2. Select the New Patient Welcome template from the Letters section of the left info panel.

3. Click the Patient Search button at the bottom to assign the letter to Ms. Ling. The patient demographics are auto-populated.

4. Confirm the auto-populated details and include any additional information needed.

5. Click the Save to Patient Record button.

EHR EXERCISES 5-3:   PATIENT EMAIL CORRESPONDENCE

*Complete the following exercise in the EHR exercises environment of SCMO.

Mora Siever (01/24/1964) had a normal left ankle x-ray last Wednesday. It is Walden-Martin policy to email patients normal results. Mora's email address is m.siever@anytown.mail. Use the Correspondence menu to create a Normal Results email for Mora.

1. Click on the Correspondence icon.

2. Select the Normal Test Results template from the Emails section of the left info panel.

3. Click the Patient Search button at the bottom to assign the letter to Mora Siever. The patient demographics will auto-populate.

4. Enter "m.siever@anytown.mail" in the To field.

5. Enter "X-ray Results" in the Subject field.

6. Confirm the auto-populated demographic details and document "left ankle x-ray" in the field with the Test Name watermark.

7. Document last Wednesday's date in the field with the Date of Service watermark.

8. Click the Send button.

Telephone Etiquette

The initial contact between the patient and the healthcare provider's office usually occurs by phone with the medical assistant. A telephone conversation, then, gives patients their first impression of the medical office. The medical assistant or staff member responsible for answering the telephone must maintain a professional and pleasant tone. It's important to remember that no matter how little you may fear for the immediate health and safety of a 7-year-old boy who has swallowed water from a goldfish bowl, to that child's mother or father, it's an emergency. Box 5-1 lists the types of phone calls a medical office is likely to receive, and Box 5-2 offers guidelines for proper **telephone etiquette.**

BOX 5-1
Common Types of Phone Calls in the Medical Office

- Appointment requests
- Inquiries from prospective patients about the practice
- Requests for medical advice from a physician or nurse
- Prescription refill requests
- Insurance and billing questions from patients
- Information requests from insurance companies
- Questions from pharmacists, medical supplies vendors, and other medical offices

---

BOX 5-2
Guidelines for Proper Telephone Etiquette

Following are some guidelines for telephone etiquette in the physician's office:
- Do not use office telephone lines for personal conversations. Keep your cell phone conversations short and private, and take such calls only while on break.
- Do not wear a Bluetooth or other cell phone earpiece during working hours.
- Greet the caller by the second ring, if possible.
- Answer the call with a professional, pleasant greeting, such as, "Good morning, Dr. Mason's office, this is Amber. How can I help you today?" The greeting should include your name so that the caller can ask for you again, if necessary, or can mention the call to another staff member (as in "I spoke to Amber yesterday about being placed on your waiting list").
- Smile as you answer the phone. Callers will hear the cheerfulness in your voice.
- Speak slowly and clearly, adjusting your volume if you know or suspect the caller has a hearing deficit.
- Obtain the caller's full name, a return phone number, and the reason for the call. Verify any spelling and contact numbers for accuracy, and summarize the reason briefly and precisely.
- If it's necessary to place the caller on hold during the call, do so only after asking the patient's permission and awaiting a response—few patients, if any, will refuse to be placed on hold when you make a polite request. Limit the hold time to less than a minute, if possible.
- Document your conversation with the caller, along with the time and date and your initials.
- To ensure all of the caller's questions have been answered, allow her or him to end the conversation.

Appointment Confirmation

According to McCauley and colleagues, the average published **show rate** for a medical practice is 58%. The younger the patient and the lower his or her income, the more likely he or she is to miss an appointment without notification. Calling a day or two ahead to confirm appointments reduces the likelihood that patients will fail to show up, thus improving continuity of care for patients, increasing practice revenues, and helping the office run more smoothly and productively. Automated systems are available for making confirmation calls, but in most small and medium-size practices, front office assistants are expected to do so. Because many people have several phone numbers, leaving messages at more than one number is advisable, provided the practice has permission from the patient to do so.

Patients who make an appointment and do not show up or do not call to cancel are considered **no-shows.** The Patient Dashboard in SCMO displays a record of appointment dates and times. The EHR produces a history of canceled appointments and no-shows for each patient. An excessive no-show rate will inhibit the functioning of the office. Patients should be encouraged to call and cancel if they can't make their appointment so that the slot can be made available to other patients. Oddly enough, medical practices might be able to learn a thing or two about no-shows from the restaurant industry, for which no-shows are a perpetual problem (see Table 5-1 and Trends and Applications 5-2).

Table 5-1 Reducing No-Shows

Restaurant Industry Tactic	Adaptation for the Medical Practice
Require diners to supply their credit card number to make a deposit that's forfeited if they don't honor the reservation.	Many medical offices now notify patients that they will be charged either a percentage of the cost of a procedure or the full cost of a visit if they skip out.
Call to remind diners of their reservation by saying, "I'm calling to confirm that you still plan to join us." Then—and here's the key—wait for an answer. Research has shown that diners who have given their word are less likely to blow off a reservation.	Medical offices can do the same—that is, call to confirm patient appointments and wait for patients to give their word that they'll either show up or call in advance to cancel.
A twist on confirming reservations is calling no-shows the following day to ask why they weren't able to come. This is a bit of a guilt trip, but it educates diners that the restaurant missed their business and was inconvenienced by their absence.	Medical offices can call patients to ask why they missed their appointments (incidentally, the most common reason is "I forgot"). Patients can be gently reminded that the physician had reserved the appointment time especially for them and can be given the option of rescheduling.
Keep callers on the phone longer. This eats up staff time, but it pays off, because diners quickly develop a personal connection with the restaurant.	Ditto. Scrap your recorded message and get a real person on the line chatting with college kids about their final exams or asking after Mrs. Millikin's new grandchild. The topic doesn't matter—showing a genuine interest in the patient's life does.
Use a waiting list and walk-ins to fill tables left open by no-shows.	Johnson and colleagues found that practices with low no-show rates are more willing to take advantage of walk-in patients and to use a waiting list to fill slots left open by no-shows and last-minute cancellations.
Stop accepting reservations altogether and seat diners on a first-come, first-served basis. This idea has worked well even at high-end restaurants like celebrity chef Rick Bayless's Frontera Grill in Chicago.	Stop accepting appointments and see patients on a total or partial walk-in basis. Some practitioners use online scheduling systems to allow patients to make their own appointments, leaving as many as two thirds of the slots open on any given day. Other practices operate in tandem a traditional appointment schedule and a fast-track room for walk-ins.

TRENDS AND APPLICATIONS 5-2

What the Restaurant Industry Can Teach Us About No-Shows

Anyone would be excused for thinking that the owner of Eddie's Steak and Chop has little in common with Edmund Newland Pierpont III, MD. But for restaurant owners and healthcare providers alike, no-shows are a continual annoyance and a financial drain. Both medical offices and restaurants routinely overbook in anticipation of no-shows. When the number of no-shows is overestimated, disgruntled patients and diners are subjected to long waits. When the number is underestimated, practices and kitchens are overstaffed. Because restaurants must keep perishables on hand, they also lose money by purchasing and prepping too much food.

Privately, restaurateurs have long bemoaned what they see as a scourge on the industry. According to the Operations and Information Management Department at the Wharton School, University of Pennsylvania, the industry-wide no-show rate in 2012 was estimated to be around 20% for big cities. The rate of absenteeism surges on Saturdays and can be as high as 40% on weekends and during special occasions, such as graduation day in a college town.

The no-show rate among medical practices, curiously enough, falls within the same range. According to a February 2013 article in the *Pittsburgh Post-Gazette,* the average

TRENDS AND APPLICATIONS 5-2—cont'd

no-show rate for urban family clinics can typically be seen between 10% and 20%. However, these statistics can vary month to month or even week to week. Unfortunately, those specialty practices that are already difficult to get into can sometimes see no-show rates of as high as 50% in a single week. The no-show rate tends to be higher among practices with a large proportion of new, self-pay, or Medicare patients. The proportion is lower among practices with a large proportion of patients 46 to 64 years old and among clinics that treat more chronically ill, rather than acutely ill, patients.

The restaurant industry has become remarkably aggressive and creative in combating truant diners. One restaurateur sued a would-be diner who reserved a four-top and failed to show. The court sided with the merchant, awarding him $200 in lost revenue plus the $400 that he'd paid a private eye to track down the malingerer. Another disciplinary tactic has been to embarrass deserters by listing their names on public reservations websites such as opentable.com. Perhaps a compassionate industry like healthcare can't borrow the most punitive of these strong-arm tactics, but many restaurant-industry solutions *are* adaptable to healthcare. A few clever ideas are listed in Table 5-1.

It is helpful to develop a script for making confirmation calls. With the implementation of technology, offices are using email and text messaging to confirm patient appointments. This script should become part of the office procedures manual. In addition to the date and time, the script might include the following points:

- A reminder that the physician has reserved this time especially for him or her
- A request to return the call to confirm the appointment or to reschedule if necessary
- A request to bring to the appointment a list of current medications because many patients receive prescriptions from several different specialists
- A reminder for the patient to check on his or her referral status if the patient's insurance company requires a referral
- A list of forms of payment the practice accepts (for example, "We now accept MasterCard and Visa for your copayment, or you can pay by cash or check if you prefer")

Paper-based offices have to pull a patient's chart a day or two ahead of time to ensure that the chart can be located and that all recent correspondence received has been filed in it. An EHR eliminates that step. All test results, referral letters, and other important clinical information will already be in the patient's EHR. However, office staff should check to make sure that the provider has reviewed these items before the patient's visit. Finally, when making the confirmation call, staff should take the opportunity to check for any billing issues or insurance questions that need to be addressed.

Occasionally patients cannot be contacted via phone prior to their appointment because the phone was disconnected, the number changed, or the number had been incorrectly entered into the EHR. In such cases staff should ask the patient to update contact information during check-in.

EHR EXERCISE 5-4:   COMPOSE A PHONE MESSAGE

*Complete the following exercise in the EHR exercises environment of SCMO.

Dr. Pericardio has called at 1:15 PM today to discuss patient Noemi Rodriguez (11/04/1971). Her echocardiogram was positive for MVP and Dr. Pericardio requests that Dr. Walden return his call when he is free. Dr. Pericardio can be reached after 4 PM today at 123-545-8912. Compose a phone message to communicate this information to Dr. Walden.

1. Select the Correspondence icon.

2. Select the Phone Message template from the left info panel.

3. Click the Patient Search button to perform a patient search and assign the phone message to Ms. Rodriguez.

4. Confirm the auto-populated details and enter any necessary information based on the case study.

5. Click the Save to Patient Record button.

EHR EXERCISE 5-5: COMPOSE A PHONE MESSAGE

*Complete the following exercise in the EHR applications environment of SCMO.

Consumer Pharmacy called at 10 AM to inform the Walden-Martin office that they have a shortage of Abilify. The pharmacy expects to get their shipment Saturday but will not be able to fill a prescription for Noemi Rodriguez (11/04/1971) until then. Compose a phone message to inform Dr. Martin of this shortage using the same workflow provided in EHR Exercise 5-4.

Secure Email

Secure email is an inexpensive, efficient system for exchanging messages through the Internet using secure **encryption technology.** This versatile means of communication has many different uses in the medical office. The office accountant may email an insurance company to obtain an authorization. The office manager may email other staff regarding changes in office procedures. One practice may email another to request a referral for a patient office visit. Other common message topics include patient orders, notification of schedule changes, and patient education. Box 5-3 offers guidelines to ensure that email correspondence reflects professionalism.

BOX 5-3
Guidelines for Sending Professional Email

Email sent from your office email account should reflect a high level of professionalism. Remember that email is a form of documentation. Accordingly, much of the email you send and receive will end up in a patient's permanent legal medical record. The following are guidelines to help you ensure that your email messages meet the highest professional standards.

- Ask yourself whether sending an email is the best way to communicate in a given situation. The tone of an email message can easily be misinterpreted, especially when addressing touchy subjects. Reread your email before sending, and consider asking a staff member for a second opinion.
- Never send an email to anyone immediately after an unpleasant incident, when you are still upset about it. If you must write it, save a draft of the message and review it when you have a cooler head. You can always send it later, but you can't take it back later.
- Triage messages as you receive them, expediting those that are urgent. You may need to refer to the patient's EHR to determine how to prioritize a message.
- Avoid the temptation to offer a diagnosis or treatment advice in response to a patient's email; leave clinical tasks to the provider.
- Use a descriptive, specific subject line (for example, Mandatory Staff Meeting, 11/15, 4:30).
- Proofread your message carefully for typographical and grammatical errors.
- Avoid using all-capital letters in the body of your message or in the subject line.
- Keep your messages brief, and use a formal but conversational style.
- Never send jokes, stories, chain letters, or other inappropriate content.
- After forwarding or replying to an email, file or archive it in the correct part of the EHR. A backlog of unfiled messages creates confusion that may lead to critical errors, such as missed test results.

Using the messaging system built in to an EHR application ensures secure delivery of email within the practice and offers a way to communicate with staff regarding confidential patient information. Providers and staff can communicate with patients via secure email using any of several commercially available HIPAA-compliant secure email services. These services also offer web hosting, spam filtering, virus protection, and related accessories, such as shared calendars and address books.

Regardless of the specific use, secure email takes the place of interoffice messages—sticky notes and the like—and postal mail, which may take days to reach its destination. However, it must be used properly to prevent the unauthorized disclosure of confidential patient information. Messages must be encrypted and sent via a secure server, and a HIPAA disclosure should be attached to each message (Figure 5-1).

Figure 5-1
A sample HIPAA email disclosure.

> *The materials in this email are private and may contain Protected Health Information (PHI). If you are not the intended recipient, be advised that any unauthorized use, disclosure, copying, distribution, or the taking of any action in reliance on the contents of this information is strictly prohibited. If you have received this email in error, please immediately notify the sender via telephone or return mail.*

✔ SECURITY CHECKPOINT 5-1

Keeping Office Email Messages Secure

- Verify the email address of the recipient to ensure your message reaches the correct person, particularly if you have trouble reading an email address handwritten on a form.
- Inform the recipient of the sensitive nature of the email.
- If you don't receive a reply to a message in which a reply was requested, follow up by phone, mail, or fax to make sure the message was received. Don't simply resend the message to the same email address.
- Do not cc messages to others unless asked to do so, and obtain authorization when necessary.
- Develop an office policy and a related patient handout specifying what types of communication may be exchanged by email, who has access to the patients' confidential email messages, what the expected response time is, whether minors may exchange email with the office, and so on.
- Remember that your email message may end up being read by recipients other than the person for whom it was intended. A good rule of thumb is never to write anything in an email message that you wouldn't write in a letter. Figure 5-2 shows a sample secure email agreement that can be adapted for an office and distributed to patients.

EHR EXERCISE 5-6:   COMPOSE A PATIENT EMAIL MESSAGE

*Complete the following exercise in the EHR exercises environment of SCMO.

Norma Washington has been waiting for the smoking cessation program to begin at Butler Hospital, and you received word today that 6-8 PM classes will start this Monday in the Lawson meeting room. Compose an email message for Ms. Washington informing her of this program. Her email address is n.washington@anytown.mail.

1. Select the Correspondence icon.

2. Select the Blank Email template from the Emails section of the left info panel.

3. Click the Patient Search button to assign the email message to Ms. Washington.

4. Confirm the auto-populated details and enter any necessary information based on the case study.

5. Click the Save to Patient Record button.

CRITICAL THINKING EXERCISE 5-3

Think of the types of messages you might document for a physician. What types of patient inquiries are appropriate and inappropriate for message documentation?

Figure 5-2

A sample secure email agreement. (Courtesy of St. Clair Pediatrics, Swansea, IL.)

St. Clair Pediatrics

Secure E-mail Agreement

Greg T. Garrison, M.D.
Jill A. Johnston, M.D.
Kevin M. Ponciroli, M.D.

E-mail us at mydocs@stclairpediatrics.com

In our continuing effort to better serve our patients and their families, we have set up an e-mail address through which you may communicate your child's protected health information with our office. It is your right to be informed about the risks of communicating via e-mail with your child's healthcare provider and about how we plan to use our secure e-mail service to maximize your child's medical management while maintaining his or her privacy as mandated by the American Health Insurance Portability and Accountability Act of 1996 (HIPAA).

Definitions for this Agreement
   User: any parent/guardian or other person given access to the e-mail address listed in this Agreement.
   Protected Health Information (PHI): information, including demographic information that may identify the patient, that relates to the past, present, or future physical or mental health of an individual.
What types of communication should be sent via e-mail?

Subjects appropriate for e-mail	Subjects not appropriate for e-mail
Prescription refills	Urgent questions regarding your child's health
Lab results	Sensitive topics such as:
Appointment requests	HIV-related issues
Referral requests	Other sexually transmitted diseases
Billing questions	Mental health issues
Requests to have forms or immunization records completed	Substance abuse issues
Non-urgent, chronic disease management questions	(These topics should be discussed with your child's physician in person.)
General feedback (positive or negative comments regarding office policies or staff)	

What are the benefits of using e-mail?
   E-mail allows quick and detailed communication with our office for non-urgent matters.
   E-mail allows retention and clarification of advice provided in clinic.
   E-mail is useful for information you would have to commit to writing if it were given to you orally.

What are the risks of using e-mail?
   E-mail is not appropriate for urgent matters or emergency situations. E-mail, by its very nature, is a delayed communication. Our e-mail is not accessed and read continuously (see "Office policies regarding e-mail" on page 2). We cannot guarantee that any particular e-mail will be read and responded to within any particular period of time.
   E-mail is sent at the touch of a button. Once sent, an e-mail message cannot be recalled or cancelled.
   Errors in transmission, regardless of the sender's caution, can occur.

What are the benefits of the secure e-mail service known as SecureSend used by St. Clair Pediatrics?
   To comply with the guidelines regarding patient and medical records privacy set forth by HIPAA, we have engaged a third-party provider to manage our secure e-mail system: Lux Scientiae (for more information on the company, please visit www.LuxSci.com). The company uses HIPAA-compliant encrypting technology (SecureSend) to ensure security of messages sent using its system. To access these messages, the User will be required to enter two passwords. The first is a User-specific password created by each User during the on-line registration of his/her e-mail address. The second is a randomly generated password included in each e-mail. This ensures that only the person registering a valid e-mail address has access to a child's PHI.
   Everyone may use this service regardless of the type of e-mail program they have (i.e., Outlook Express, Internet Explorer, etc.). Message links embedded in the body of each e-mail direct you to a secure internet website. NOTE: You **do** need internet access to view secure e-mail messages.
   In general, e-mail can be circulated, forwarded, and broadcast to unintended recipients. Using the SecureSend web portal, you can only send an e-mail to those accounts set up through Lux Scientiae's SecureSend (which, for us, is mydocs@stclairpediatrics.com).

Figure 5-2, cont'd

St. Clair Pediatrics	**Secure E-mail Agreement**	Greg T. Garrison, M.D. Jill A. Johnston, M.D. Kevin M. Ponciroli, M.D.

Office policies regarding e-mail

Response time: E-mail will be checked only during normal office hours, 4 times per day (or more). We will make every effort to respond to e-mails within 24 hours. An e-mail sent after 12:00 PM on Friday will not receive a response until the following Monday.

E-mail access: E-mail will be managed primarily by the clinical and nursing staff. All staff members will have password-protected access to the general e-mail service. Pertinent questions and concerns will be discussed with your child's physician before the staff responds.

E-mail responses: If the question you submit can be responded to in a short and concise manner, the staff will reply via e-mail. However, for questions that require a more detailed response, the staff will contact you via telephone. Please make sure to include your phone number on all e-mails you send to us.

Office security: All desktop workstations in the office are equipped with password-protected screen savers.

E-mail security: We will not forward patient-identifiable information to a third party without your express permission. We will not use registered e-mail addresses in marketing schemes or give out your address to third parties.

Your teenager will also be allowed to use this service: Any child over the age of 13 may sign himself/herself up for the e-mail service. This allows your child to continue to communicate with his/her physician openly, honestly, and confidentially about all subject matters.

E-mail directions

E-mail must be concise: Please limit each e-mail message to one issue. This allows us to maximize message triage efficiency. Please schedule an appointment for your child if the issue is too complex or sensitive to discuss via e-mail.

All e-mails must include: The e-mail's subject line should include the reason for your e-mail followed by your child's name (i.e., "Refill Request, Joe Smith"). The body of the e-mail should include all information pertinent to your request, as well as the phone number(s) where you can be reached in case the office staff needs to speak with you.

Before transmitting the e-mail: Please double-check the message and any attachments to verify that no unintended information is included.

E-mail communications will become a part of your child's medical record: All pertinent e-mails will be printed and/or filed in your child's medical record.

Signing up and using the Service

Step 1: Read this Agreement and complete page 3. This Agreement will only be accepted in person at our office. **IMPORTANT:** We will only reply to e-mails from Users that have submitted this Agreement in person.

Step 2: Log on to securesend.stclairpediatrics.com (a link can also be found on our main web page, www.stclairpediatrics.com).

Step 3: Set up your account by clicking on "Register your email address for secure sending." Enter your name, e-mail address, and password. This password is the one you will use to log onto securesend.stclairpediatrics.com with your e-mail address. You then need to create a security question and password. These will be used to access a secure e-mail sent you by mydocs@stclairpediatrics.com.

To send an e-mail: Log onto securesend.stclairpediatrics.com with your e-mail address and password. You can then "Send a New Secure Message" to mydocs@stclairpediatrics.com by clicking "Compose."

To access an e-mail sent to you from mydocs@stclairpediatrics.com: The e-mail you receive will contain the line: "Click here to access your message." After clicking the link, you will be taken to a web portal, which will request two passwords. The first is the correct response to the security question you created during account registration. The second is specific to the e-mail sent to you and can be located in the body of the e-mail. You will then be taken to the actual e-mail sent to you by mydocs@stclairpediatrics.com.

IMPORTANT: The only way to ensure the information you send is secure is by logging onto securesend.stclairpediatrics.com. **We have set up our account so that we only receive e-mails sent through this website.**

Compare the efficiency of electronic messaging systems to that of a paper-based system. Some offices use a time and date stamp to log incoming messages. Most of us recall—or perhaps are still using—those pink "While You Were Out" memo pads for transcribing phone messages. Messaging in a paper-based office might also consist of scrawling a few facts on thin little slips of perforated carbon paper no bigger than a dry-cleaning ticket—and just as easy to misplace.

These loose message slips are then placed in a bin or a tray on the physician's desk. If the provider needs to view the patient's chart in order to respond, the chart must be pulled. The staff has little way of knowing whether the physician has read a message, reviewed a lab result, or returned a call. Sometimes the only clue that the physician hasn't is a third or fourth phone call from an increasingly irate patient. Once the request has been dealt with, a message is filed in the patient's paper chart. This small piece of carbon paper may be the only permanent record of the call and its content.

Paper or electronic, it is best to follow some simple guidelines to ensure the patient care is upheld while taking a message:

1. Document the patient name, date of birth, and phone number on the message.
2. Document the date and time of the call.
3. Document all instructions and conversations with the patient.
4. Document the name or initials of the person taking or returning the call on the message.
5. Once the message is complete and the documentation is sufficient, save the message to the patient's chart.

Faxing

A **fax machine** is a device that encodes documents in order to transmit them over telephone lines. The fax, like email, enables quicker message transmission than traditional mail. However, it poses several security and integrity risks:

1. Faxes can be misdirected because of human error or technical glitches.
2. The recipient of a fax cannot be verified because anyone can pick up the printed document if the machine is placed in an unsecure location.
3. It is difficult to verify that all pages were received.
4. You can mitigate these risks by following some commonsense guidelines:
5. Inform the recipient prior to sending any confidential patient information so that it can be retrieved immediately.
6. Use a cover sheet when sending a fax (Figure 5-3). The cover sheet should include the sender's contact information, a confidentiality disclaimer, and recipient information.
7. Follow up with the intended recipient to ensure that the message was received.
8. Document the date and time, and initial the faxed information to create a paper trail.
9. File the completed cover sheet in the patient's chart.

An attractive alternative to faxing is to send and receive secure fax transmissions via secure email. This system for encrypting fax transmissions and sending them via email makes a fax machine obsolete, eliminating the hassles of changing toner and clearing paper jams. It also saves the practice the expense of maintaining a fax machine and paying for an additional phone line. The system works by electronically recording fax transmissions and storing them as PDF files. If a hard copy is needed, these faxes can be printed, just like regular faxes.

MANAGING ELECTRONIC HEALTH RECORDS

The EHR is only as good as its security. It must be monitored daily to ensure the program's integrity. EHRs that are not closely monitored are at risk of vandalism by computer hackers and are vulnerable to destruction by natural disaster or other means. If records are damaged or destroyed, patient care could be compromised.

Maintaining the EHR is the responsibility of the entire office, and each person may have specific responsibilities. The providers, office manager, and system administrator determine which major software updates are necessary and when the changes will be made. Staff members (medical assistants, nurses, billing staff, and receptionists) must maintain patient confidentiality and may be responsible for backing up the EHR. Training sessions should be conducted not only during the process of implementing the EHR but also periodically throughout the year. Additional training sessions will restore proficiency in forgotten applications, build competency in executing complex functions, and inform users about new EHR capabilities.

Figure 5-3

Example of a fax cover letter.

Medical Facsimile Cover Sheet

Date: _____

TO

Name	
Phone	
Fax	

FROM

Name	
Signature	
Phone	
Fax	

Patient Name	
Identifier	
Medical Record Number	

Reason for Release	

Information Released	

Total Pages _____

IMPORTANT: This facsimile transmission contains confidential information, some or all of which may be protected health information as defined by the federal Health Information Portability and Accountability Act (HIPAA) Privacy Rule. This transmission is intended for the exclusive use of the individual or entity to whom it is addressed and may contain information that is proprietary, privileged, confidential, and/or exempt from disclosure under applicable law. If you are not the intended recipient (or an employee or agent responsible for delivering this facsimile transmission to the intended recipient), you are hereby notified that any disclosure, dissemination, distribution, or copying of this information is strictly prohibited and may be subject to legal restriction or sanction. Please notify the sender by telephone (number listed above) to arrange the return or destruction of the information and all copies.

Eliminating Duplicate Charts

The EHR should be a complete collection of a patient's health information; however, sometimes a duplicate patient chart is created in error. Perhaps the patient's last name changed due to marriage, or the patient was set up as a new patient when in fact the patient had been seen before. This duplication creates a serious problem because it divides the patient information between two charts. To avoid this, the medical office staff must ask pointed questions during the patient interview:

1. Ask whether the patient has ever been seen by the practice before. If so, use the already established patient EHR. Regardless of whether patients believe they are new to the office, always perform a patient search before creating a new record.
2. Ask established patients whether they have had a name change.

3. Always set up the patient EHR account using the name listed on the insurance card. Claims submitted with names that do not precisely match that on the insurance card may be denied for payment.

Purging Patient Records

Patient health records can be classified into three different groups: active, inactive, and closed. *Active records* are those of patients who have been seen within the past 3 years (see Chapter 2). These records are easily accessed and used frequently. *Inactive records* are those of patients who have not been seen by any provider in the medical office within the past 3 years. *Closed records* are those of patients who have terminated their relationship with the medical office—some have moved away, others have been asked to leave the medical office because of bad debt or failure to follow physician advice, and some have died.

HIPAA law states that the patient health record must be kept permanently, not that it must remain in the office. When **purging**, closed records are separated from active ones and stored elsewhere. Some closed records are placed on CDs or computer hard drives or maintained in inactive cloud space by the EHR vendor. Paper charts may be scanned into microfilm.

As discussed in Chapter 2, the retention period is the amount of time, by law, that patient records must be maintained by the medical office. Retention periods vary from state to state. Patient health records must be maintained for evidence of patient care in the event a lawsuit is filed.

CRITICAL THINKING EXERCISE 5-5

Sandra Trotter presents to the receptionist today asking for a copy of her immunization records. Upon investigation, the receptionist finds that it has been 7 years since Ms. Trotter has been seen by any of the physicians in the practice. Inactive and closed records are stored at a separate location and can take up to 2 weeks to get out of storage. How can the receptionist explain this delay to Ms. Trotter, who is insisting that she leave with her records?

Backing Up the Electronic Health Record

With the use of paper-based records, backing up patient records consists of little more than storing charts in filing cabinets that are locked at the end of the day. Charts are at risk of damage from wear and tear, weather, and accidents (such as the occasional spilled cup of coffee). Paper records can be irrecoverably damaged or lost in a fire or flood.

EHRs eliminate this concern if the records are backed up at a secondary, offsite location. When the software is working, the medical office can run smoothly and efficiently. But no matter what precautions the medical office takes, trouble can still arise. For example, the power may be lost during severe weather, disabling computers and other electronic equipment (including the EHR). Virus attacks, hardware or software failures, and simple human error can bring a medical office to a standstill.

Some medical offices store a charged portable laptop computer in the medical office. A laptop can run on battery power for a short time until the electricity is restored. Then the device should be recharged for future emergency use. Some offices may revert to written documentation while the power is off and then input the data once the software is running again. Caution should be taken, however, because rewriting documentation increases the risk of error. It's good practice to input only the data you gathered yourself and not information that a coworker gathered. This kind of backtracking can cost the practice thousands of dollars in paid overtime for office staff.

Backup takes place at a minimum of once daily to every 15 minutes or even as often as every keystroke. It's usually the job responsibility of one or two reliable workers, or the

EHR vendor may conduct routine backups. Although having offsite copies of patients' charts is an advantage to patients, security must be monitored closely. Patient confidentiality and security must remain as much of a priority for the backup copies as it is for the primary EHR systems in the medical office. For this reason, backup copies should be stored in a remote location, such as a bank vault, or maintained by a separate entity, such as the EHR vendor. The EHR vendor may provide a data recovery package that can guarantee data backup or recovery and virus protection. An EHR vendor based as software as a service (SAAS) (see Chapter 4) will remotely provide backups online to minimize the risk of lost information.

The medical office must, by law, have a written backup and recovery plan in place (see Chapter 3). This detailed document should be stored in the office policies and procedures manual and be easily accessible. This plan should outline what constitutes an emergency and provide contact information for restoring the EHR (if the vendor is responsible for doing so), the location of the backup copy, instructions for managing patients while the software is down, and plans for inputting the data once the software becomes functional again.

CALENDAR

Traditionally patient appointments have been maintained using paper desk calendars or appointment books—and, of course, the appearance is unorganized. Scribbled names and scratched-out, overwritten, or double-booked appointments make the schedule hard to decipher. It's often difficult to reschedule appointments and find available time slots. Another disadvantage is that only one person can use the appointment book at a time.

This system has the medical assistant flipping back and forth, searching for availability within a specified time slot while perhaps one or two coworkers wait to schedule other patients. This haphazard method can cause stress for both medical assistants and patients. In addition, poor scheduling leads to longer patient wait times, a key factor in determining patient satisfaction. Patients should be seen within 5 to 10 minutes of arrival, but absolutely no more than 15 minutes of wait time should occur.

In the medical office, an electronic appointment book is the key to efficient time management. Several users can access the electronic appointment book at once. Patient appointment sheets can be printed out daily so that the physicians, medical assistants, nurses, and receptionists are all aware of the patient load for the day. Patients can be easily rescheduled, and appointment availability can be searched based on patient preferences.

When using an electronic appointment book, the medical assistant simply enters the appointment criteria—say, a weekday between 11:30 and 1:00—and reserves specific examination rooms (and therefore, be sure appropriate equipment is available) for the patients. At the same time, coworkers can be setting up appointments for other patients or viewing provider appointments.

When an appointment is scheduled, the patient's demographic information is auto-populated in the appointment book. This allows the healthcare staff to verify insurance eligibility, confirm appointment dates, or edit patient information.

Calendar Views

In a paper system there are only two ways of viewing an appointment book: open or closed. The SCMO scheduling system offers many different **views,** accessible from the blue tabs on the left side of the screen: Calendar View, Exam Room View, and Provider View (Figure 5-4). Users can also view a patient's next scheduled appointment using the Search field (Figure 5-5).

Scheduling in SCMO is done by clicking on the orange Add Appointment button from the Calendar View (Figure 5-6) or by double-clicking within the calendar. The New Appointment box appears (Figure 5-7). SCMO allows the user to enter three different types of appointments.

1. Patient Appointments—new and established patient visits with any of the three providers in the office (Dr. Walden, Dr. Martin, or Jean Burke)

Figure 5-4
Calendar View tabs.

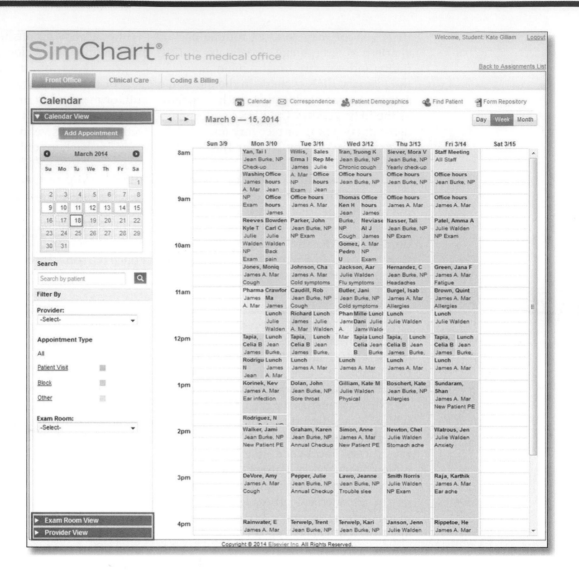

Figure 5-5
Search field.

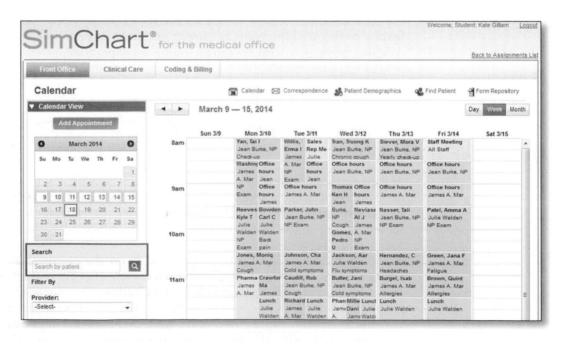

Figure 5-6
Add Appointment
button.

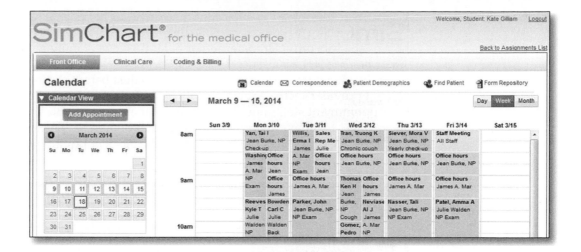

Figure 5-7
New Appointment box.

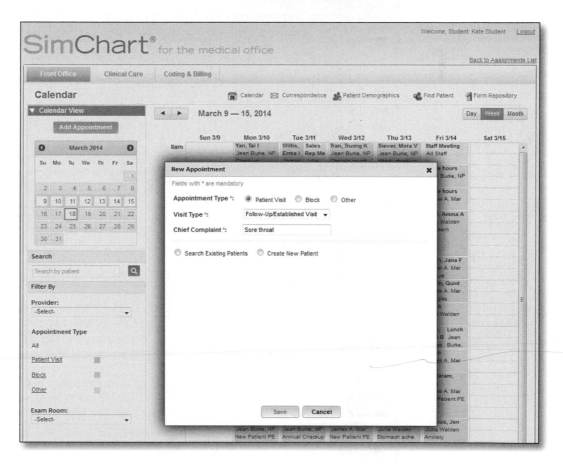

2. Block Appointments—indicates times that a provider is unavailable due to lunch, out-of-office time, office hours, or holidays
3. Other Appointments—time for staff, sales, and pharmaceutical meetings

Block an Appointment Time

Appointment slots might be blocked for a variety of reasons, such as the following:
1. To account for routine days off, such as holidays
2. To schedule provider vacations, business travel, or personal time off. Some offices block out more and more time during the last several days before a trip and then open up the slots for urgent care patients as the need arises. During the provider's

absence, they may also block out time on his or her partners' schedules so that they can cover urgent care visits while the physician is away.

3. To schedule provider maternity or paternity leave, family medical leave, sick leave, or other leaves of absence
4. To block out time before and after lunch or just before closing, ensuring that the staff and providers actually get to eat lunch and perhaps leave the office by quitting time

Appointment slots should be blocked out as soon as you know the time has become unavailable. Holidays and other office closings should be blocked at the beginning of the year. To block out time in the calendar, use the block appointment type.

EHR EXERCISE 5-7:   SCHEDULE A PATIENT APPOINTMENT

*Complete the following exercises in the EHR exercises environment of SCMO.

Susannah Ling (01/02/1973) calls Walden-Martin to set up a new patient appointment with Dr. Martin next Wednesday at 10 AM. Dr. Martin requires 30 minutes for appointments with new patients. Schedule an appointment for Ms. Ling.

1. Within the Front Office, Calendar, click the Add Appointment button.

2. Within the New Appointment window, select Patient Visit as the appointment type.

3. Select New Patient Visit as the visit type.

4. Document New Patient PE as the Chief Complaint.

5. Susannah Ling was added as a Walden-Martin patient in Chapter 2, so select the Search Existing Patient radio button and click the Save button to search for Susannah's record.

6. Select James A. Martin, MD, as the provider.

7. Use the calendar picker to select next Wednesday as the appointment date.

8. Select a start time of 10:00 AM and an end time of 10:30 AM.

9. Click the Save button. A confirmation message will appear and the appointment will be displayed on the calendar.

Chase Murray called complaining of a rash on his lower extremities. He would like to see Dr. Martin but isn't available until next Wednesday at 1 PM. Dr. Martin requires 15 minutes for urgent office visits. Schedule an appointment for Mr. Murray, using exam room 4.

Prison guard Miles Green was bitten by the drug-sniffing canine during training this morning and will need sutures. Schedule an urgent appointment with Jean Burke, NP for 30 minutes at 4 PM.

Al Neviaser needs to schedule a follow-up appointment with Dr. Walden to check his high blood pressure. Mr. Neviaser is available next Wednesday at 11 AM. Dr. Walden requires 15 minutes for follow-up appointments and likes to perform these types of visits in exam room 6.

EHR EXERCISE 5-8:   EDIT AN APPOINTMENT

*Complete the following exercise in the EHR exercises environment of SCMO.

Susannah Ling calls back and states that her car will not start. She would like to reschedule her appointment. Move her appointment to this Friday at 10 AM.

1. Click on Ms. Ling's existing appointment on the calendar.

2. Within the Saved Appointment window, use the calendar picker to select this Friday as the appointment date.

3. Click the Save button. A confirmation message will appear and the appointment will be updated on the calendar.

EHR EXERCISE 5-9:   DELETE A PATIENT APPOINTMENT

*Complete the following exercise in the EHR exercises environment of SCMO.

Chase Murray calls Walden-Martin later in the day and reports that his rash turned out to be dry skin. Cancel his appointment.

1. Click on Mr. Murray's appointment on the calendar.

2. Change the status to Canceled using the Status drop-down at the bottom of the Saved Appointment window.

3. Document the reason for cancellation and click the Save button.

4. A confirmation message will appear and the appointment will be removed from the calendar.

EHR EXERCISE 5-10:   BLOCK TIME FOR A STAFF MEETING

*Complete the following exercise in the EHR exercises environment of SCMO.

Dr. Walden and Dr. Martin want to schedule a staff meeting to discuss opening a new laboratory, new uniform requirements, and professionalism. An hour-long time slot is open this Friday at 3 PM. Coffee and water will be provided. Reserve the meeting room for this meeting and arrange for coffee and water to be provided.

1. Click the Add Appointment button. Select Other as the appointment type.

2. Select Staff Meeting as the Other Type.

3. Select Meeting Room as the Location.

4. Select All Staff as the Attendees.

5. Use the calendar picker to select this Friday as the meeting date.

6. Select a start time of 3 PM and an end time of 4 PM.

7. Document the agenda in the Description field as "Discussion topics: New laboratory opening, new uniforms, and professionalism. Coffee and water provided."

8. Click the Save button. A confirmation message will appear and the meeting will be displayed on the calendar.

EHR EXERCISE 5-11:   BLOCK OUT-OF-OFFICE APPOINTMENTS

*Complete the following exercise in the EHR exercises environment of SCMO.

Jean Burke, NP, is attending a training seminar for wound treatment on Monday from 9 AM to 12 PM and will not be available for patient appointments during that time. Block this time for Jean Burke, NP.

1. Click the Add Appointment button. Select Block as the appointment type.

2. Select Out-of-office as the Block type.

3. Select Jean Burke, NP, to specify who this blocked time is for.

4. Because this time will be spent in the office, no location is needed.

5. Use the calendar picker to select Monday as the meeting date.

6. Select a start time of 9 AM and an end time of 12 PM.

7. Document "Wound treatment training" as the Description.

8. Click the Save button. A confirmation message will appear and this time will be blocked on Jean Burke, NP's, calendar.

Double-Booking

Double-booking may be done for any or all of the following reasons:
1. The practice expects a certain number of no-shows.
2. The practice expects certain patients to arrive early and others to arrive late, which staggers their appointment times even though the schedule shows them as being double-booked. This is an especially good scheduling strategy if patients' appointments are expected to be brief.
3. The two patients being booked in the same slot are being seen for different reasons that require different rooms and resources. For example, one patient might be scheduled for an annual physical. While the medical assistant is taking his or her vitals, another patient might be having a mole removed for evaluation by a pathologist.
4. A patient with an urgent medical problem, such as acute fever, needs to be accommodated.

You can insert a second appointment at a time you choose, or you can search for an appropriate slot by date and time, type of visit, or other criteria by following the same step for inserting a patient appointment described earlier. Keep in mind that physicians will have specific preferences as to when double-booking may occur. For example, some may only allow double-booking during the first appointment of the day, whereas others prefer double-booking slots directly before their lunch hour.

The goal of efficient scheduling is to optimize **patient flow** through the practice. An efficient flow requires an accurate estimation of patient volume. Scheduling must be realistic given the provider's general pace. Habitual overbooking and ineffective scheduling techniques will lengthen wait times and leave providers alternately swamped or idle.

WAITING ROOM

A patient's path through the practice begins in the waiting room. And let's be honest—no one likes waiting rooms. The name alone implies you will be there for a while. They tend to be populated by fussy children, folks with wracking coughs, and—at the very least—outdated, dog-eared magazines. Fellow patients either whisper to one another or shout on cell phones. Usually a vapid talk show or soap drones overhead, and you begin to doze off with a copy of *Modern Kayaker* or *Today in Foreign Affairs*.

It's part of the medical assistant's job to ensure that the waiting room is well lit, clean, and safe. Because well patients may be exposed to sick ones while waiting to see the physician, keeping the waiting room clean is particularly important. Although toys can help keep small children occupied, caution should be taken to ensure that they don't serve as a means of passing bacteria and viruses from one child to another and that they do not pose a choking hazard. The toys must be cleaned and disinfected daily, and broken toys should be thrown away.

Reading material in the medical office should be current, and not include potentially offensive topics. It's best to avoid magazines or brochures on religion or partisan politics. Commercial solicitations for products or services not approved by the U.S. Food and Drug Administration (FDA), such as herbal products and questionable treatment regimens, are also inappropriate.

Instead, use the waiting room as an opportunity to promote healthy lifestyles. Patients may not otherwise have a chance to read about consumer health, nutrition, disease prevention, health maintenance, fitness, and a positive self-image. Information on these topics should be offered instead of the usual assortment of sports, celebrity gossip, and news magazines, which patients can pick up elsewhere. Many modern medical offices are installing kiosks at which patients can complete registration forms or learn how to log into their new patient portal. Others offer interactive applications as patient education tools. Fish tanks are also popular additions to waiting rooms because of their calming presence and are less of a nuisance than television.

CHAPTER SUMMARY

- The front office assistant must be well-trained, versatile, and positive toward patients, providers, and other staff. Front office duties include greeting patients on the telephone and in person, taking accurate phone messages, creating and managing an EHR for each patient, scheduling appointments, and generating correspondence.

- Good communication among providers, patients, and staff improves patients' confidence in their care, increases their satisfaction with the medical practice, makes healthcare personnel feel better about their jobs, and prevents many medical errors.

- Proper telephone etiquette includes answering calls promptly, using a professional greeting, asking for the caller's full name and reason for calling, writing down a return phone number, documenting the conversation, and allowing the caller to terminate the conversation.

- Secure email is an inexpensive, efficient system for exchanging messages through the Internet using a secure encryption technology.

- A fax machine is a device that encrypts and decodes documents so that they can be quickly transmitted over telephone lines. Fax transmissions can also be sent via secure email.

- Patient health records can be classified into three different groups: active, inactive, and closed. Inactive or closed medical records are purged when the retention period expires or when the patient transfers to a different practice or dies. Patients' health information stored in the EHR must be protected from destruction by computer hackers, natural disasters, terrorist attacks, and other untoward events.

- SCMO allows the medical assistant to schedule, block, or change appointments. Using an EHR to organize appointments makes it easy to search for available slots, edit or delete appointments, keep track of patient no-shows, and double-book as needed. It is part of the medical assistant's job to ensure that the waiting room is well lit, clean, and safe. The wait time for the patient should not exceed 15 minutes, and time waiting should be used to promote health and wellness.

CHAPTER REVIEW ACTIVITIES

Key Terms Review

Match the term in column A to the definition in column B.

1. Appointment slot
2. Double-booking
3. Encryption technology
4. Secure fax
5. No-show
6. Patient flow
7. Purging
8. Retention
9. Secure email
10. Show rate
11. Telephone etiquette
12. Views
13. Waiting room

a. The first stop in a patient's path through the medical office

b. A system capable of transmitting an encrypted message and storing it in coded format until it is retrieved by the recipient via a secure web link

c. The period of time patient records must, by law, be maintained by the medical office

d. The percentage of patients in a practice who arrive for appointments as scheduled or call in advance to cancel or reschedule

e. Giving two or more patients the same appointment time with the same provider

f. The process of separating inactive patient health records from active ones

g. A polite, helpful response and respectful manner toward callers

h. A patient who makes an appointment and neither shows up nor calls to cancel

i. A period of time reserved for a patient to see a healthcare provider

j. Different ways of displaying the same or similar information on a computer screen, usually with increasing or decreasing detail

k. A fax transmission sent via secure email

l. A system that keeps data secure by converting it into an unreadable code during transmission and then unencrypting the information when it reaches the recipient

m. A product of accurately estimated patient volume, a consistent provider pace, and efficient scheduling practices

True/False

Indicate whether the statement is true or false.

1. _____You should avoid apologizing to patients because doing so constitutes an admission that the practice has made a mistake.

2. _____The HIPAA Privacy Rule allows medical practices and other covered entities to disclose some healthcare information via email, fax, or phone without specific patient authorization, provided reasonable precautions are taken to protect privacy.

3. _____Use of a script is a helpful way for patients to understand that the physician has reserved specific time for them.

4. _____HIPAA-compliant secure email services may also offer web hosting services, spam filtering, virus protection, and related accessories, such as shared calendars and address books.

5. _____Always set up the patient EHR account using the name listed on the insurance or ID card.

6. _____Several users can access the electronic appointment book at once.

7. _____EHR users should find the scheduling view that works best for their office and ask the administrator to program it in permanently.

8. _____Appointment slots should be blocked out for trips, holidays, or out-of-office time using the Block Appointment type.

Workplace Applications

Using the knowledge you obtained from the chapter, complete the following activities.

1. You are interested in updating the look and feel of the office waiting room. Create a layout to fit seating for 10 patients. What elements will you include to make the space productive and pleasant for the patient experience?

2. Chase Murray is having difficulty sleeping and would like to schedule an appointment with Dr. Martin next Tuesday at 9 AM. Use exam room 2 to schedule this 30-minute appointment.

3. CPR recertification training will be available for the entire staff on November 1 from noon to 4 PM in the meeting room. All office attendees who plan to attend must notify Marta at extension 30. Block this time on the calendar.

4. Schedule a wellness exam for Tai Yan (04/07/1956) with Dr. Walden next Monday at 9 AM. The appointment will last 30 minutes and take place in exam room 4.

5. Truong Tran (05/30/1991) needs to discuss recent episodes of depression with Jean Burke, NP. Next Monday at 1 PM will work best for him. Schedule this 30-minute office visit in exam room 7.

6. This Saturday, the Walden-Martin office will be purging health records of patients who have not been seen in the past 3 years. Use the memorandum email template in the Correspondence menu to invite available employees to assist in this process from 8 AM to 2 PM. Employees will be paid overtime and lunch will be provided. Those interested should notify Marta at extension 30. Use the office email WMstaff@waldenmartin.com to complete this communication.

7. Maria Hernandez calls the office today for her daughter, Casey Hernandez (10/08/2000), who was exposed to poison oak while playing in the woods behind their house this weekend. She now has a red rash on her left calf that is seeping clear liquid. Casey complains that the rash is very itchy. Ms. Hernandez is working today and unable to bring Casey in. She wonders if Jean Burke, NP, could call in a prescription to help with the rash. Casey is not allergic to any medications. The Hernandez family uses Waltman's Family Pharmacy at 123-445-3200. Ms. Hernandez's work number is 123-445-5122. Compose a phone message for Jean Burke, NP, to communicate this question.

EHR in Review

Your chance to keep past skills current. Try these activities covering previous content.

1. Interview a fellow classmate to register him or her as a new patient in SCMO. Remember to first perform a patient search within Patient Demographics to avoid creating a duplicate record. After confirming that your classmate is not registered in the system, use the Add Patient button to begin the patient registration process.

2. Noemi Rodriguez needs a copy of her electrocardiogram (ECG) from January 2014 sent to Dr. Pericardio for review prior to her appointment. Prepare a Medical Records Release

allowing Dr. Martin to send this record. The release will expire in 30 days. Dr. Pericardio is located at 455 Heart Valve Way, Anytown, AL 45582.

3. Chris Miller, father and guarantor of patient Daniel Miller, has new contact information. His cell phone number is 123-555-6363 and his work number at the auto shop is 123-540-4774. Update this contact information in the Guarantor tab of Daniel's Patient Demographics.

BIBLIOGRAPHY

Anderson, R. T., Camacho, F. T., & Balkrishnan, R. (2007). Willing to wait? The influence of patient wait time on satisfaction with primary care. *BMC Health Services Research*, 7, 31.

Balasubramanian, V. (2007). *Are reservations recommended?* Kellogg Insight. Kellogg School of Management: Chicago. Available at: http://insight.kellogg.northwestern.edu/index.php/Kellogg/article/are_reservations_recommended. Accessed 26.01.09.

Baxter, S., Farrell, K., Brown, C., et al. (2008). Where have all the copy letters gone? A review of current practice in professional-patient correspondence. *Patient Educ Couns.* 1(2):259-64.

Burke, L., & Weill, B. (2009). *Information technology for the health professions* (3rd ed.). Upper Saddle River, NJ: Pearson.

Chung, M. K. (2002). Tuning up your patient schedule. *AAFP's Family Practice Management*, January. Available at: www.aafp.org/fpm/20020100/41tuni.html. Accessed 28.01.09.

Dimick, C. (2007). Selling physicians on EHRs: Illustrating the benefits to care, the importance of data. *Journal of American Health Information Management Association*, June, 46–48.

Fordney, M. T. (2006). *Insurance handbook for the medical office* (9th ed.). St. Louis: Elsevier.

Grace, S. (2007). Technology: Backing up to move forward. *Physician's Practice*, June. Available at: www.physicianspractice.com/display/article/1462168/1588630?pageNumber=3. Accessed 11.06.11.

Grzybowski, D. (2008). A plan for paper in the transition to electronic document management. *Journal of American Health Information Management Association*, May. Available at: http://library.ahima.org/xpedio/groups/public/documents/ahima/bok1_038089.hcsp?dDocName=bok1_038089. Accessed 11.06.11.

Huff, C. (2008). Diagnosis: Doctor's office rebellion. *American Way Magazine*, 7, 14–18.

Krishna Y.I., and Damato B.E. (2005). Patient attitudes to receiving copies of outpatient clinic letters from the ocular oncologist to the referring ophthalmologist and GP. *Eye (Lond).* 19(11):1200-4.

Johnson, B. J., Mold, J. W., & Pontious, J. M. (2007). Reduction and management of no-shows by family medicine residency practice exemplars. *Annals of Family Medicine*, 5(6), 14–18.

Levinson, W., Roter, D. L., Mullooly, J. P., et al. (1997). Physician-patient communication: The relationship with malpractice claims among primary care physicians and surgeons. *Journal of the American Medical Association*, 277(7),

Martin, Z. (2008). Be prepared. *Health Data Management*, 534–539.

McCauley, J., Jenckes, M. W., Atwood, M., et al. (2000). Does a computerized telephone reminder system improve medical appointment show rate in inner city, general internal medicine, managed care practices? *Academy for Health Services Research and Health Policy*. Available at: www.healthdatamanagement.com/issues/2008_45/25627-1.html?zkPrintable=true. Accessed 11.06.11.

National Restaurant Association. (2000). *How to reduce no-shows*. National Restaurant Association How-to Series. Available at: www.restaurant.org/business/howto/noshows.cfm. Accessed 26.1.09.

Oh, J., & Su, X. (2012). *Pricing restaurant reservations: Dealing with no-shows*. Available at: https://opimweb.wharton.upenn.edu/linkservid/3AB9C6AC-E733-B5F7-F509202003B1FFFA/showMeta/0/. Accessed 20.3.14.

Rinehart-Thompson, L. A. (2008). Record retention practices among the nation's "most wired" hospitals. *Perspectives in Health Information Management*, 5(Summer), 8.

Toland, B. (2013). *No-shows cost health care system billions: But clinics, hospitals may be as much to blame as patients*. Available at: www.post-gazette.com/business/businessnews/2013/02/24/No-shows-cost-health-care-system-billions/stories/201302240381. Accessed 20.3.14.

Young, A., & Proctor, D. (2012). *Kinn's the medical assistant: An applied learning approach* (12th ed.). St. Louis: Mosby.

chapter 6

Clinical Use of the Electronic Health Record

Chapter Outline

Commission on Accreditation of Allied Health Education Programs (CAAHEP) Competencies

1. Document patient care.
2. Differentiate between subjective and objective information.
3. Compose professional/business letters.

Chapter Objectives

1. Describe the benefits of documentation in the electronic health record (EHR).
2. Explain the role of speech recognition software in medical documentation, and describe the benefits of the technology.
3. List the components of the medical, surgical, family, and social history.
4. Explain how the chief complaint and history of the present illness relate to each another.
5. Enter allergies, medications, and intolerances into an EHR.
6. Discuss what components of a patient's vaccination history should be included in the chart.
7. Describe how to record vital signs and anthropometric measurements in the EHR.
8. Outline the process many physicians use for constructing a progress note.

Key Terms

acute condition An illness or injury that is episodic (e.g., a seizure), has a sudden onset (such as a broken bone), is of limited duration (e.g., bronchitis), and generally responds well to prompt medical attention.

anthropometric measurements Measurements of height, weight, and size used to compare the relative proportions of the human body in health and illness.

chronic condition An illness that persists for a prolonged time (typically 3 months or longer) and requires periodic follow-up with a healthcare provider, regardless of whether the condition has a sudden or gradual onset.

e-visit An evaluation and management service provided by a physician or other qualified health professional to an established patient using a web-based or similar electronic-based communication network for a single patient encounter that occurs over safe, secure, online communication systems.

high-alert medication A medication that poses a heightened risk of injury or death when administered improperly.

history of the present illness (HPI) Details about the duration, time, location, severity, context, associated signs and symptoms, quality, and modifying factors related to the patient's illness.

medication reconciliation The process of comparing the medication list in the patient's EHR with the patient's self-report of the medications he or she has been taking.

objective Readily seen, perceived, or measured by the clinician, not only by the patient.

PFSH An abbreviation for past (medical), family, and social history.

postural blood pressure (posturals) Blood pressure readings taken in different positions: recumbent, sitting, or standing.

review of systems (ROS) An organized inventory of each organ system, completed as part of the initial patient interview to pinpoint any unusual findings in the patient's history.

speech recognition A technology that converts speech into text.

subjective Perceived only by the patient and not evident to or measurable by the clinician.

DOCUMENTATION IN THE ELECTRONIC HEALTH RECORD

"If it hasn't been documented, it never happened" is the mantra drilled into the heads of medical, nursing, and medical assisting students everywhere. It's the healthcare profession's equivalent of "What happens in Vegas stays in Vegas—if no one has a camera phone handy."

The electronic health record (EHR) is used to record, for instance, patient history, chief complaint, vital signs, allergies, patient education, medication lists, and test results. This documentation helps the provider achieve a high standard of care. Each member of the healthcare team, at various times, will need to review or edit information in the EHR. It's important that the information added be accurate and directly reflects the actions taken during the patient encounter. Falsifying patient records is illegal and can lead to termination, civil penalties, or criminal prosecution.

Documentation is the most important responsibility of all members of the medical office. How does documentation facilitate healthcare delivery? Let us count the ways. Documentation does the following:

- Makes diagnosis and treatment more efficient and more likely to be effective
- Promotes patient safety and reduces medical errors by conveying critical information to other healthcare providers
- Serves as a risk management function by providing evidence of communication between practitioner and patient and by illustrating the quality of care delivered
- Provides evidence of care delivery for third-party payer reimbursement
- In an EHR, proper documentation allows related items, such as health history, progress notes, patient letters, and patient instructions, to be linked and easily accessed.

It's not enough, though, for documentation just to be present and accounted for. It must be thorough and tidy, too. The fastest way to burst a defense attorney's bubble is to hand over a shipshape EHR in which progress notes are cogently written, laboratory report and imaging studies have been reviewed and signed, and findings and follow-up have been neatly documented. Trends and Applications 6-1 discusses tips for ensuring proper documentation. This advice can be shared with providers and staff alike as part of a comprehensive compliance plan.

TRENDS AND APPLICATIONS 6-1

Tips for Street-Smart Documentation in the EHR

Composition instructors are fond of reminding students that poor writing rarely masks a brilliant insight lying just below the surface; on the contrary, jumbled sentences probably indicate muddled thinking. Clarify your ideas, and your writing will shine. Likewise, excellent documentation and high-quality care are closely related. Juries leap to conclusions about physicians whose records are sketchy, and for good reason—because it's probably true.

Good documentation prevents many errors and shows evidence of quality care. Here are some tips to improve documentation practices in your office:

1. Record all findings, both positive and negative. This includes the patient's progress since the last visit, especially if he or she is being seen for a chronic illness. Note the patient's response or lack of response to treatment, including any side effects. The documentation need not be exhaustive, but concise documentation must hit all the salient points.
2. Include evidence of clinical decision making, unless it is clearly implied by the findings. Document treatment and follow-up, even if a wait-and-see approach is taken. Evidence of medical decision making is doubly important from a legal standpoint when the provider decides that it's wisest to do nothing.
3. Review and sign notes, reports, and letters. Leaving such documents unsigned suggests that the provider did not have a complete picture of the patient's health status at the time he or she formulated the treatment plan.
4. Identify the patient's risk factors. Use the extensive history and relevant clinical information stored in the EHR to find the patient's soft spots. Note any conditions in the patient's family history, social history, and lifestyle or social habits that could predispose him or her toward developing certain conditions.
5. Make sure the CPT and ICD-10 codes selected are consistent with the narrative documentation. Any discrepancies could make the documentation suspect.
6. Pay special attention to prescription documentation. Refer to the list of Error-Prone Abbreviations, Symbols, and Dose Designations issued by the Institute of Safe Medication Practices (ISMP) until you know it. Use the substitutions the ISMP suggests. Avoid trailing zeros (as in "25.0"), which can make 25 mg look like 250, and naked decimal points (as in .25), which can make 0.25 mg look like 25.

Does an EHR improve clinical documentation? According to a study by Rouf and colleagues, the answer is yes. They surveyed third-year medical students working in outpatient clinics, and 69% agreed that using an EHR improved their documentation. In particular, they reported that the prompts built into the system led them to ask more questions when taking a patient's history. Half of the participants said they were also more likely to review and sign patients' tests in an EHR than in a paper chart.

Voice Recognition

As discussed in Chapter 1, an EHR can make the problem of physicians' notoriously poor penmanship a moot point. Providers who wish to do so can document patient encounters by dictating into the medical record with the aid of **speech recognition** software, a technology that converts speech into text as the provider speaks into a microphone. This kind of documentation eliminates the need for a staff member to file physician documentation into a paper chart or to transcribe a tape recording into the record.

The speech recognition used in medical dictation is a different application of the same technology used in call routing (as in "Press or say 'one' now"). It's even used in the avionics systems of high-performance aircraft to allow pilots to carry out tasks such as setting radio frequencies and changing displays on cockpit gauges. It has other applications, too, ranging from computer gaming to court reporting.

Software for the medical office incorporates a complete dictionary of medical terminology and abbreviations. The physician is able to dictate patient notes directly into the patient health record. This technology offers several advantages, including the following:

- Allows the user to work hands-free
- Eliminates the problem of misplaced or misfiled patient notes
- Decreases the rate of transcription mistakes
- Lowers the cost of transcription
- Reduces the amount of time necessary to complete documentation
- Increases the overall quality of patient care

According to a white paper by National City Corp., which finances many small medical offices, transcription costs about 11 cents per line, and an average patient encounter generates about 35 lines. That may not sound like much, but in a small clinic with two physicians, two nurse practitioners, and a load of about 14,000 visits per year, the total can swell to more than $50,000.

Speech recognition capability is available as an add-on to EHR systems. It's compatible with Dragon Naturally Speaking, a popular speech recognition program that works best when the user speaks in an animated tone.

Using Dragon, you can open any of its menus. An extensive set of voice commands is used to accomplish that task you'd normally do with the keyboard, such as "Insert a comma" and "Scratch that" to delete the last thing you said. Dragon is voice recognition software that uses acoustic data to recognize your way of pronouncing things, so that the right spelling will pop up if you say "tomato" and someone else in your office says "tomahto." These files also store customized terms, acronyms, and abbreviations you add to the Dragon vocabulary.

CRITICAL THINKING EXERCISE 6-1

In addition to speech recognition capabilities, what advantages does electronic documentation in an EHR offer over handwritten documentation in a paper chart?

Documenting Remote Patient-Provider Encounters

Telephone Documentation

Can a practitioner document care for a patient he or she hasn't seen that day? The answer, of course, is yes. Physicians must document all prescription refills called in or emailed to pharmacies in response to patients' phone requests. And nearly every day they document medical advice offered during calls with anxious parents of feverish children or with patients having abdominal pain or back spasms or panic attacks.

In fact, Katz and colleagues reviewed 32 telephone-related malpractice cases and found that faulty documentation was a key factor in 88% of the errors that led to the lawsuits. These mistakes had devastating physical consequences for patients and led to an average payout of $512,000 per case for insurance companies. According to a study by Schmitt, 80% of cases are dropped if the practice is able to show, by way of excellent documentation, that a reasonable standard of care was met.

E-Visits

Advancing technology has changed not just the way patient encounters are documented, but also the way patients are seen by a physician. Physicians may not make house calls anymore, but they make mouse calls. The American Academy of Family Physicians (AAFP) defines an **e-visit** (also termed *web visit* or *online consultation*) as an evaluation and management service provided by a physician or other qualified health professional to an established patient using a web-based or similar electronic-based communication network for a single patient encounter that occurs over a safe, secure, online communication system.

E-visits give the patient a way to be "seen" by the physician without leaving his or her home or office. The patient saves travel time, decreases lost work hours, and could decrease long-term healthcare costs.

E-visits are the most successful in monitoring chronic disease. For example, diabetes, hypertension, and asthma can be monitored via e-visits on a regular basis. More and more insurance companies are beginning to pay for e-visits, reimbursing an estimated $25 to $35 per visit. Medicare, however, doesn't currently cover this service. Insurance providers who cover e-visits do require the patient to pay a regular office copayment.

The AAFP suggests the following guidelines for e-visits:

- E-visits should be offered only to established patients.
- The patient must initiate the process and agree to the terms of service. These terms include the provider's charges and privacy policy.
- Electronic communication must occur over a HIPAA-compliant online connection.
- The practitioner must appropriately document the e-visits as he or she would any other visit.
- The provider should define the time period during which the e-visit will be completed.

CRITICAL THINKING EXERCISE 6-2

In your opinion, are there any healthcare problems that should not be treated via e-visit? Why are e-visits not recommended for new patients?

CLINICAL DOCUMENTATION IN THE PATIENT RECORD

In the Who Documents in the Medical Record? section of the first chapter, you learned that many staff members within the physician's office contribute to the medical record. After the receptionist records the basic data about the patient, the next documenter is typically the medical assistant. After placing the patient in an examination room, this clinical staff member asks the patient questions related to his or her reason(s) for seeing the provider (chief complaint), the history of the chief complaint, current symptoms, previous medical history including similar injuries or illnesses, current prescriptions and over-the-counter medications, medication allergies, and any other nursing observations. In addition, the clinical staff member records the patient's height, weight, and vital signs, including blood pressure, pulse, temperature, and respiration rate.

Patient Encounter

Every patient visit must be documented as evidence of care. In SimChart for the Medical Office (SCMO), the patient visit is called an *encounter,* and there are three types: Comprehensive Visit, Office Visit, and Phone Consultation. The Encounters grid in the Patient Dashboard displays the encounter type, creation date, and status of existing encounters (Figure 6-1). Users can view, edit, or create new documentation in any past encounter by clicking on the encounter in the Type column.

Documenting patient care within an encounter allows the user to enter all clinical information pertaining to the date of service. To create a new patient encounter in SCMO:
1. Click the tab for the Clinical Care module.
2. Perform a Patient Search. Selecting the patient will display the Patient Dashboard (see Chapter 2).
3. Select a New Encounter type from the left Info Panel.
4. Specify the date and visit type in the Create New Encounter window.
5. Click the Save button to add the patient encounter.

Figure 6-1
Encounter Info panel.

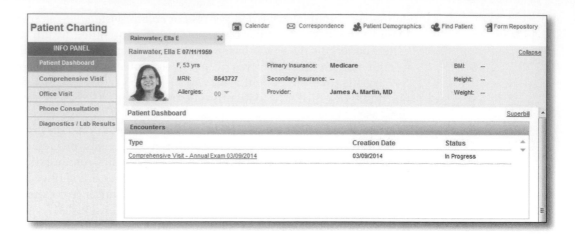

6. Clinical documentation for that encounter can begin. Users land within the Allergy record section by default but can navigate to other sections using the Record drop-down menu.

EHR EXERCISE 6-1:   CREATE AN ENCOUNTER

*Complete the following exercise in the EHR exercises environment of SCMO.
   Susannah Ling (01/02/1973) arrives for her new patient appointment today. Create a New Patient Office Visit encounter in SCMO.

1. Click the tab for the Clinical Care module.

2. Perform a patient search for Susannah Ling and confirm her date of birth.

3. Select Comprehensive Visit from the left Info Panel.

4. Use today's date as the default, and select New Patient Visit from the Visit Type drop-down menu.

5. Click the Save button.

ALLERGIES

Patients may have many different types of allergies or intolerances, including environmental, seasonal, and contact allergies, along with allergies to certain medications and allergies to, or intolerance of, certain foods. Knowing about a patient's allergies is important in providing proper patient care. Each patient should be asked to verify his or her allergies at the start of each visit or encounter, before medication is administered or other treatment is given, and before any medical procedures are performed. For example, before performing venipuncture, the medical assistant must ask whether the patient is allergic to latex or adhesives.

The patient's EHR should be updated when the allergy list changes. The reaction to an allergen should also be documented with the EHR. Allergic reactions range from urticaria (hives) to pruritus (itching) to edema (swelling) to dyspnea (difficulty breathing) and chest pain. Edema of the airway may be severe enough to cause respiratory failure, so allergies must be taken seriously.

The allergies record section is the default landing page upon entering a patient encounter within SCMO. The medical assistant can verify existing allergies, document that a patient has no known allergies, and add or edit allergies to the patient record. Most clinical records in SCMO start by clicking the Add button, and the allergy record is no exception (Figure 6-2). Allergens can be selected from a preexisting allergy database using the drop-down menu or typed directly into the field. This flexibility provides both structured and unstructured data entry.

Figure 6-2
Add Allergy button.

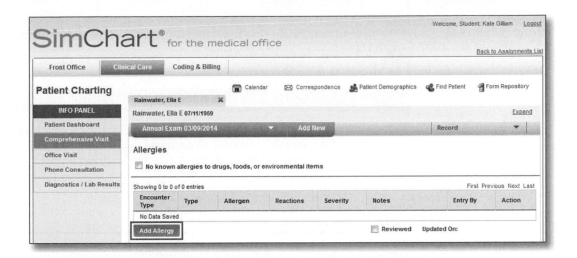

EHR EXERCISE 6-2:   DOCUMENT PATIENT ALLERGIES

*Complete the following exercise in the EHR exercises environment of SCMO.

During the patient interview, Susannah Ling (01/02/1973) explains she has an allergy to ciprofloxacin tablets. This medication causes a reaction of itching and hives. Ms. Ling states the reaction seems be to moderate. Document Ms. Ling's allergy in her record.

If you are not already in the patient's encounter, remember to enter the Comprehensive Visit, New Patient encounter in order to document in this record.

1. Within the Allergy record section, click the Add Allergy button. An Add Allergy window will appear.

2. Select the Medication radio button in the Allergy Type field.

3. Document "Ciprofloxacin Tablet (Cipro)" in the Allergen field (Figure 6-3).

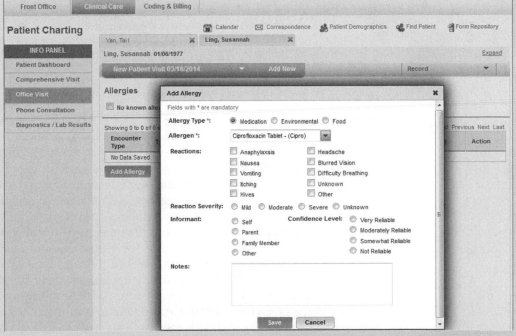

Figure 6-3   Add Allergy box.

4. Select the Itching and Hives check boxes to indicate the reactions.

5. Select the Moderate radio button to indicate the reaction severity.

6. Select the Self radio button to indicate that the patient is reporting her own allergy.

7. Select the Very Reliable radio button to indicate the confidence level.

8. Click Save to add ciprofloxacin to the patient's allergy grid.

EHR EXERCISE 6-3:   DOCUMENTING ENVIRONMENTAL ALLERGIES

*Complete the following exercise in the EHR exercises environment of SCMO.

During the patient interview, Susannah Ling (01/02/1973) expresses an allergy to foam rubber which results in severe headaches and blurred vision. Use the previous workflow to document this environmental allergy in Ms. Ling's record.

PATIENT HISTORY

We're all familiar with those new patient forms you have to fill out when you change physicians. You're handed a clipboard with a pen chained to it and asked to check yes or no on what seems like several dozen boxes. This form is part of the patient history, which includes past (medical), family, and social history **(PFSH).** A new patient history is likely to include a comprehensive and detailed **review of systems (ROS),** whereas an established patient history is focused on a particular problem or condition.

All components of the history are important in treating and caring for patients and must be recorded in the EHR. The practitioner or other interviewer should take his or her time and consider each of the patient's responses carefully to ensure that all areas have been covered. Traditionally offices have mailed a questionnaire to patients and ask them to complete it before their first visit. More recently, health history forms can be completed through web-based patient portals, thus reducing paperwork lost, necessary information forgotten at home, or illegible handwriting. Allowing patients to complete these forms at home gives them time to recall all important parts of their medical background in a comfortable setting. Any positive (yes) responses to the ROS questions should prompt more specific follow-up questions.

CRITICAL THINKING EXERCISE 6-3

Do you think patients should receive paperwork, such as a review of systems, before their appointments? How can the implementation of technology and patient portals improve the process of gathering data?

MEDICAL AND SURGICAL HISTORY

A new patient must also be interviewed, usually by both a medical assistant and the practitioner, to gather as much health information as possible. This information is useful in determining a patient's risk for disease and in diagnosing, monitoring, and treating medical conditions. It includes a review of past illnesses, surgeries, hospitalizations, and treatment. During the medical history, the interviewer should also ask about drug allergies, take down a list of the patient's current medications and dosages, record the patient's vaccination history, and note his or her history of exposure to communicable diseases, such as hepatitis and tuberculosis, if known.

Other questions asked during the medical history depend on the patient's individual needs. For example, the provider may ask an excessively thin young woman about her eating habits and whether she's had any recent weight loss to determine whether she may have an eating or thyroid disorder. An older man may be asked whether he's experiencing any urologic problems, such as a need to urinate with excessive urgency or frequency.

Surgical history should include a record of any adverse reactions to anesthesia, a note of any other complications, the date of surgery, and the name of the institution at which it was performed.

SCMO organizes health history into three tabs (Figure 6-4):

- Medical History—Past Medical History (PMH), Past Hospitalizations, and Past Surgeries.

Figure 6-4
Health History tabs.

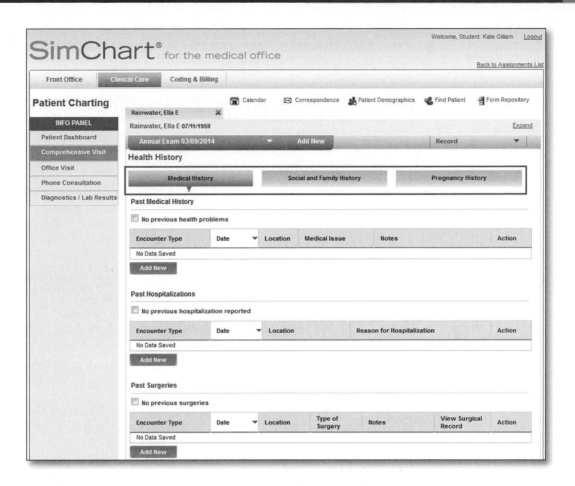

- Social and Family History—Safety in the Home, Paternal and Maternal Health History, marital status, employment, tobacco, drug and alcohol use, exercise habits, nutrition, and dental history
- Pregnancy History—Previous Pregnancies and significant reproductive history for female patients

Once in a patient encounter, select Health History from the Record drop-down menu. New history items can be added to each tab using the orange Add New buttons.

EHR EXERCISE 6-4:   DOCUMENT HEALTH HISTORY

*Complete the following exercise in the EHR exercises environment of SCMO.

During the patient interview at the Walden-Martin office today, Susannah Ling (01/02/1973) states that she has a history of iron deficiency anemia and anxiety. Her past surgeries include a rhinoplasty at Plastic Surgery Associates on November 1, 2013, and an appendectomy at Butler Ambulatory Center on November 19, 1999. She has no previous hospitalizations. Ms. Ling lives with her husband Russell, age 39, daughter Ella, age 3, and son Gunner, age 1. Ella was conceived naturally. Gestation was 39 weeks and Ms. Ling was in labor for 16 hours before a vaginal delivery with no complications. Stadol was the only medication administered. Ella weighed 6 pounds, 7 ounces. Gunner was also conceived naturally. Gestation was 40 weeks and Ms. Ling was in labor for 12 hours before a vaginal delivery with acute mastitis after delivery, which is now resolved. Ms. Ling received an epidural. Gunner weighed 8 pounds, 0 ounces.

Ms. Ling states that she feels safe at home. She is satisfied with her job as a florist. She drinks a glass of red wine occasionally with dinner but has never used tobacco products or illegal drugs. She does not exercise regularly or follow a special diet. She consumes two cups of coffee each day. She has not had any abortions or miscarriages. Her last dental visit was February 20, 2014, with Dr. Bonnett. Her father, Bert, is 64 and has hypertension and atrial fibrillation. Her mother, Shelly, is 66 and has a history of left breast cancer, which is in remission.

Use the Health History record to document in each of the three history tabs. Be sure to save your work when finished.

1. Within the Medical History tab, click the Add button beneath the Past Medical History grid.

2. In the Add Past Medical History window, using today's date, document "Walden-Martin Family Practice" as the location and "Iron deficiency anemia" as the medical issue. Click the Save button and repeat this workflow to document Ms. Ling's past medical history of anxiety.

3. Click the Add button beneath the Past Surgeries section.

4. In the Add Past Surgeries window, document "November 1, 2013" as the date, "Plastic Surgery Associates" as the location, and "Rhinoplasty" as the type of surgery. Click the Save button and repeat this workflow to document Ms. Ling's appendectomy.

5. Within the Social and Family History tab, click the Add button beneath the Family History grid.

6. In the Add Family History window, document "Russell" as the name, "39" as the age, and "Husband" as the relationship. Click the Save button and repeat this workflow to add Ella and Gunner.

7. Select the Yes radio button to indicate that Ms. Ling does feel safe in her home.

8. Click the Add button beneath the Paternal section.

9. In the Add Paternal Family Member window, document "Father" as the relationship, "64" as the age, and "Hypertension and atrial fibrillation" as current medical conditions. Click the Save button and repeat this workflow for Ms. Ling's mother in the Maternal section.

10. Use the Parents Marital Status drop-down menu to indicate that Ms. Ling's parents are married.

11. Use the Employment drop-down menu to indicate that Ms. Ling is satisfied with her job and document "Florist" in the Comments field.

12. Within the Tobacco/Drugs/Alcohol section, select the Occasionally radio button to indicate how frequently Ms. Ling drinks alcohol and document "Red wine" in the Comments field.

13. Select the Never radio buttons to indicate Ms. Ling's usage regarding tobacco and illegal substances.

14. Within the Activities/Exposures/Habits section, select the No radio button to indicate that Ms. Ling does not exercise regularly.

15. Within the Nutrition section, select the No radio button to indicate that Ms. Ling does not follow a special diet and consumes caffeine. Document "2 cups a day" to indicate the amount of caffeine Ms. Ling consumes.

16. Within the Dental History section, document Ms. Ling's last exam as "February 20, 2014" and dentist as "Dr. Bonnett."

17. Within the Pregnancy History tab, document "2" in the Gravida and Para fields to indicate the patients has had 2 pregnancies and 2 live births.

18. Document "0" in the Abortions and Miscarriage fields.

19. Click the Add button below the Previous Pregnancies grid to document Ella's birth history.

20. Document "3 years" to indicate that the pregnancy was 3 years ago.

21. Document "Natural" in the Conception Method field.

22. Document "39 weeks" in the Gestational Weeks field.

23. Document "16 hours" in the Duration of Labor field.

24. Document "6 pounds, 7 ounces" in the Birth Weight field.

25. Select the Female radio button to indicate the sex.

26. Document "Vaginal" in the Type of Delivery field.

27. Document "Stadol only" in the Anesthesia field.

28. Select the No radio button to indicate that this was not a preterm labor.

29. Document "None" in the Complications field and click the Save button.

30. Click the Add New button to document Gunner's birth history.

31. Document "1 year" to indicate that the pregnancy was 1 year ago.

32. Document "Natural" in the Conception Method field.

33. Document "40 weeks" in the Gestational Weeks field.

34. Document "12 hours" in the Duration of Labor field.

35. Document "8 pounds, 0 ounces" in the Birth Weight field.

36. Select the Male radio button to indicate the sex.

37. Document "Vaginal" in the Type of Delivery field.

38. Document "Epidural" in the Anesthesia field.

39. Select the No radio button to indicate that this was not a preterm labor.

40. Document "Mastitis after delivery, now resolved" in the Complications field and click the Save button.

CHIEF COMPLAINT

Patients come to the physician's office for many reasons. Some require medication refills. Others want to get their insurance and billing questions answered. However, the majority of patients are seeking medical care for acute or chronic problems. **Acute conditions** occur suddenly and are usually severe but of brief duration. Sinusitis, urinary tract infections (UTIs), and fever are examples of acute conditions. Congestive heart disease, asthma, and multiple sclerosis (MS) are examples of chronic conditions. **Chronic conditions** are those that persist over a long time or are recurrent. Regardless of the patient's reason for seeking healthcare services, the medical assistant must determine the chief complaint.

The chief complaint (CC, or cc) is the patient's main reason for seeking medical care. Many providers now prefer to use the term *chief concern* because *complaint* implies that the patient is quarrelsome or just plain whiny. **The CC should be recorded using the patient's own words.**

Sometimes a patient has more than one reason for seeing the physician. It is important to know this when the patient makes the appointment to ensure that the appropriate amount of time has been set aside for the visit. In some cases, if the patient has additional, emergent issues, the physician may ask the patient to schedule another visit to accommodate the amount of time needed to address the less pressing concerns. Seeing patients for multiple problems during a brief appointment slot tends to back up appointments for the remainder of the day.

Pain Scale

As part of the **history of the present illness (HPI),** the severity of the patient's condition will be assessed. The severity or intensity of the patient's pain is commonly documented on a pain scale, or the *fifth vital sign* as it is sometimes called. The patient is asked to qualify his or her pain on a scale of 1 to 10, with 10 being the worst. This, again, is based on the patient's words, just like the CC, and can be broken down to better determine how uncomfortable the patient is. For example, a value between 1 and 3 is mild pain, between 4 and 7 is moderate, and between 8 and 10 is severe pain. Other methods for determining the severity or level of discomfort for a patient include visual analog scales, in which the patient marks a spot on a

10-cm line, or the Wong-Baker FACES Pain Rating Scale used by young children. The pain scale reported by the patient is an important indicator to determine whether the patient's reported pain is consistent with the provider's physical examination findings for level of pain.

EHR EXERCISE 6-5: DOCUMENT CHIEF COMPLAINT

*Complete the following exercise in the EHR exercises environment of SCMO.

A dog bit Miles Green (08/30/1983) about 3 hours ago and Jean Burke, NP, is examining the 5-cm laceration on his left anterior palm. Mr. Green states a severity of 5 on a scale of 1 to 10 and describes the pain as throbbing and constant. Advil has helped the pain a little bit. During the review of systems, Mr. Green denies fever, chills, sweats, and fatigue, but admits to joint swelling and injury. He reports no other signs and symptoms. Document the chief complaint in the patient record.

1. Click the tab for the Clinical Care module.

2. Perform a patient search for Miles Green and confirm his date of birth.

3. Select Office Visit from the left Info Panel.

4. Use today's date as the default, and select Urgent Visit from the Visit Type drop-down menu.

5. Click the Save button.

6. Document the reason for Mr. Green's visit in the Chief Complaint field (Figure 6-5).

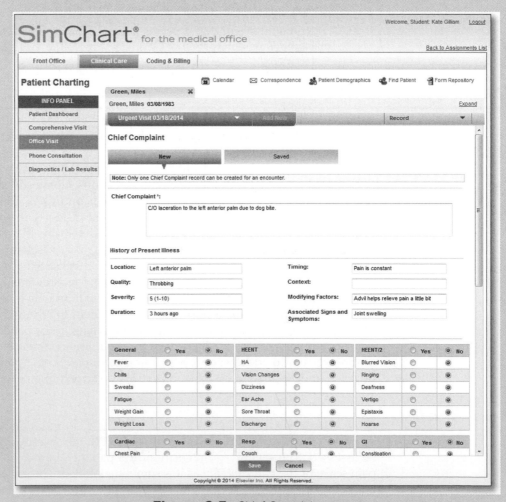

Figure 6-5 Chief Complaint record.

7. Document symptoms associated with the chief complaint in the History of Present Illness section.

8. Within the Review of Systems section, select the No radio buttons for fever, chills, and fatigue. Select the Yes radio buttons for joint swelling and injury.

9. Document your name in the Entry By field and click the Save button.

PROBLEM LIST

Managing patient healthcare can be tedious. There are several elements and layers to managing a patient's case, and the amount of data to review can be overwhelming for even the most organized physician. EHR systems make this process manageable by providing a centralized location for a summary of a patient's acute and chronic conditions called the Problem List. Meaningful use has recognized Problem Lists as one of the core objectives (see Chapter 4) for improvement of patient care. According to the American Health Information Management Association (AHIMA), the Problem Lists provide the following benefits:

■ Allow customized care by identifying the most significant health concerns
■ Help identify "disease specific populations" through data analysis
■ Help evaluate standard measures for specific providers and healthcare organizations
■ May identify patients for possible research studies

EHR EXERCISE 6-6:   MAINTAINING PROBLEM LIST

*Complete the following exercise in the EHR exercises environment of SCMO.
    Dr. Martin diagnosed Susannah Ling (01/02/1973) as having iron deficiency anemia and anxiety. Add this diagnosis to Ms. Ling's Problem List.

1. Click the tab for the Clinical Care module.

2. Perform a patient search for Susannah Ling and confirm her date of birth.

3. Select the correct encounter from Ms. Ling's Patient Dashboard.

4. Select Problem List from the Record drop-down menu and click the Add button.

5. Select "Anemia, iron deficiency" as the diagnosis.

6. Select the ICD-10 Code radio button and document "D50.0" as the code.

7. Document the date identified using the calendar picker.

8. Select the Active radio button to indicate that this is a current diagnosis.

9. Click the Save button. Ms. Ling's Problem List will update to reflect her diagnosis of iron deficiency anemia (Figure 6-6).

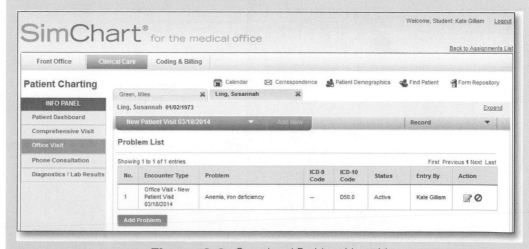

Figure 6-6 Completed Problem List grid.

10. Click the Add button and repeat this workflow to document Ms. Ling's anxiety, using ICD-10 code F41.1.

MEDICATIONS

Most patients, particularly those who are elderly or chronically ill, take multiple medications that may be prescribed by several physicians and filled at more than one pharmacy. Given this complexity, it's critical to make sure the medication list in the EHR is current. Any prescribed medications, over-the-counter (OTC) medications, and supplements the patient takes should be documented. Providers participating in meaningful use are required to report data on "maintaining an active medication list." Patients do not always remember their medications; after all, medications tend to look the same. Therefore, as part of the appointment confirmation, remind patients to bring a copy of their medications to the appointment.

EHR EXERCISE 6-7: DOCUMENTATION OF MEDICATIONS

*Complete the following exercise in the EHR exercises environment of SCMO.

Susannah Ling (01/02/1973) states she is taking alprazolam XR 0.5 mg by mouth once daily, as needed for anxiety. Her daily supplements include vitamins A, D, and C by mouth with Iron OTC, an iron supplement for iron deficiency anemia. She started taking these medications 1 year ago. Document these medications in Ms. Ling's record.

1. Within the encounter, select Medications from the Record drop-down.

2. Within the Prescription Medications tab, click the Add button.

3. Within the Add Prescription Medication window (Figure 6-7), document "Alprazolam extended release tablet (Xanax XR)" in the Medication field or select it from the drop-down.

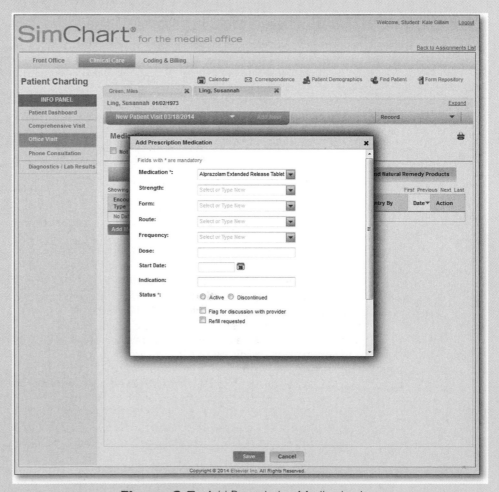

Figure 6-7 Add Prescription Medication box.

4. Select 0.5 mg from the Strength drop-down.

5. Select Tablet ER from the Form drop-down.

6. Select Oral from the Route drop-down.

7. Select Daily from the Frequency drop-down.

8. Select the start date using the calendar picker.

9. Select the Active radio button to indicate the status of the medication.

10. Click the Save button to update Ms. Ling's Medication record.

Repeat this workflow within the Over-the-Counter Products tab to document the rest of Ms. Ling's medications.

TRENDS AND APPLICATIONS 6-2

Preventing Medication Errors in the EHR

Researchers have long known that nearly two thirds of hospital records contain at least one medication error. An estimated 1 million medication errors occur each year, contributing to 7000 deaths. On average there is one medication error every day for every inpatient. In addition, pediatric patients have a threefold greater risk than adult patients of being seriously injured when a medication mistake is made.

Pharmacist Kathleen Orrico wanted to know whether the EHR systems of ambulatory care providers were any more likely to be accurate than hospital records. To find out she compared EHR medication lists against lists developed by nurses who conducted comprehensive telephone interviews with patients, which were presumably more accurate because most patients would have had access to their actual prescription bottles during phone calls taken at home. Indeed, Orrico found an average of 2.7 errors on each patient's electronic medication list.

Orrico then tried to categorize the errors by type to identify areas for quality improvement. The most common kind of discrepancy was a discontinuation (i.e., about 70% of the errors represented medications listed but no longer being taken by the patient). Omission of a multivitamin was considered an error and represented 27% of the errors attributed to patients.

The errors were classified as either patient generated, such as failure to report an OTC medication, or "system" generated, which Orrico defined as the provider's failure to update the medication list. (This euphemism may spare physicians' feelings, but it's perhaps a bit misleading in an article that also refers to electronic records systems.) Eighty percent of the errors were categorized as system generated, including failure to note the date of discontinuation for medications prescribed for a limited duration, such as antibiotics.

The Institute for Healthcare Improvement and The Joint Commission recommend that physicians do **medication reconciliation** at each visit to reduce medication errors and adverse events such as allergic reactions. Medication reconciliation is also part of the stage 1 menu set measures for meaningful use incentive. The objective requires eligible providers who receive a patient from another setting of care or provider of care should perform medication checks. This is simply a long-winded way of saying that the provider or a medical assistant should go over the patient's medications with him or her to make sure the list is accurate and current. Patients, too, must be accountable by bringing to each visit a list of their current medications and dosages. The list can be given not just to the patient's general practitioner but also to specialists, nurses, medical assistants, pharmacists, and other healthcare professionals who have a role in their care.

The following are some questions to ask patients when reconciling medications in the EHR:

■ Inquire not just about patients' prescriptions but also about their OTC medications and about dietary supplements, such as herbal products and vitamins.

TRENDS AND APPLICATIONS 5-1—cont'd

- Ask patients whether any specialist physicians or allied health practitioners, such as chiropractors, have prescribed any medications for them.
- If the patient has trouble understanding English, find out whether he or she would like an interpreter to facilitate the reconciliation process.
- Ask patients whether they ever break or cut their medication tablets; the dosage on the label is not accurate if the patient routinely breaks the tablets in half.
- Be sure to ask about oral contraceptives in female patients of childbearing age because some patients don't consider birth control pills to be medications.
- Pay special attention to verifying the dosage of high-alert medications, such as anticoagulants (blood thinners), insulin, and narcotics.

Providers, with the help of medical assistants, should document all medications, dosages, and other relevant information. The reason that a patient stops taking a specific medication should also be recorded. Perhaps the patient was taking a lipid-lowering medication that had to be discontinued because of leg cramping. Documenting such information can be used to speed insurance drug approvals, or it may remind the physician that the patient generally cannot tolerate a specific classification of drugs. As you read in the Trends and Applications 6-2 in the EHR box, it is also very important to record any OTC medications that the patient is taking, including any dietary supplements or other herbal products or vitamins. (Table 6-1 lists common prescription abbreviations.)

Table 6-1 Common Medication Prescribing Abbreviations

Abbreviation	Spelled out	Meaning
a.c.	ante cibum	Before meals
ATC	around the clock	Around the clock
b.i.d.	bis in die	Twice a day
gt.	gutta	A drop
m.d.u.	more dicto utendus	To be used as directed
NMT	not more than	Not more than
p.c.	post cibum	After meals
PO	per os	By mouth
p.r.n.	pro re nata	As needed
q3h	quaque 3 hora	Every 3 hours
q.i.d.	quater in die	Four times a day
S.A.	secundum artum	Use your judgment
sig.	signa	To write
SL	sublingually	Under the tongue
stat.	statim	Immediately
Tab	tabella	Tablet
t.d.s.	ter die sumendum	Three times a day
t.i.d.	ter in die	Three times a day
TPN	total parenteral nutrition	Nutrition administered via a nongastrointestinal route
troche	trochiscus	Lozenge
u.d.	ut dictum	As directed

IMMUNIZATION HISTORY

Immunizations protect people against infections caused by harmful microorganisms. Although we generally think of immunizations as being for children, some are recommended for adults as well (Table 6-2). Immunizations are required in various situations. For example, children must meet certain standards before starting school. Healthcare workers and others working in high-risk environments must have a hepatitis B immunization.

Table 6-2 *Recommended Adult Immunization Schedule, by Vaccine and Age Group*

Vaccine	Age Group					
	19-21 years	22-26 years	27-49 years	50-59 years	60-64 years	≥65 years
Influenza*	←1 dose annually→					
Tetanus, diphtheria, pertussis (Td/Tdap)*	Substitute one-time dose of Tdap for Td booster; then boost with Td every 10 yr					
Varicella*	←2 doses→					
Human papillomavirus (HPV), female*	←3 doses→					
Human papillomavirus (HPV), male*	←3	doses→				
Zoster					←1 dose→	
Measles, mumps, rubella (MMR)*	←1 or 2 doses→					
Pneumococcal 13-valent conjugate (PCV13)*	←1 dose→					
Pneumococcal polysaccharide (PPSV23)	←1 or 2 doses→					←1 dose→
Meningococcal*	←1 or more doses→					
Hepatitis A*	←2 doses→					
Hepatitis B*	←3 doses→					
Haemophilus influenza type b (Hib)*	←1 or 3 doses→					

☐ For all persons in this category who meet the age requirements and who lack documentation of vaccination or have no evidence of previous infection; zoster vaccine recommended regardless of prior episode of zoster.

▨ Recommended if some other risk factor is present (e.g., on the basis of medical, occupational, lifestyle, or other indication)

☐ No recommendation

*Covered by the Vaccine Injury Compensation Program.

Modified from Centers for Disease Control and Prevention. (2014). *Recommended adult immunization schedule, by vaccine and age group.* Available at: www.cdc.gov/vaccines/schedules/hcp/imz/adult.html. Accessed 20.3.14.

A tetanus vaccine should be given every 10 years, or less for those with open wound sites. The EHR can keep a running record of these vaccinations and is thus a good tool for tracking a patient's immunization history. Items documented within immunizations include:

- Name of immunization
- Date given
- Name of person administering the immunization
- Date immunization is updated (if necessary)
- Location of injection
- Category
- Manufacturer
- Type
- Expiration date
- Lot number

Documenting these details will assist the physician in the event of an adverse patient reaction or a recall from the manufacturer.

In order to maximize the physician's time with the patient, the medical assistant will want to gather some basic information about the patient's medical history. The physician will go into the patient's history in greater detail during the physician's face time with the patient. The clinical decision support functionality helps focus the medical assistant's questions to the presenting problems. In all cases, the medical assistant will want to know whether the patient has any significant medical conditions. In the case of an illness, like a cough, the medical assistant will want a brief review of the patient's ears, nose, and throat. If the patient presents with a musculoskeletal issue, the medical assistant will be presented with medical history related to previous surgeries on the affected body part or previous injuries in addition to whether the patient has any arthritis, joint problems, muscle pain or stiffness, or tendinitis.

EHR EXERCISE 6-8:   VACCINE AUTHORIZATION FORM

*Complete the following exercise in the EHR exercises environment of SCMO.

Dr. Martin ordered an influenza vaccine for Susannah Ling (01/02/1973) today. During the interview with the patient, Susannah denies illness or high fever. She does not have an allergy to chicken or eggs. She has not had any allergic reactions to injections before. Before Ms. Ling receives her influenza vaccine, prepare a vaccine authorization form for her to sign.

1.   Within the Form Repository, select the Vaccine Authorization (Figure 6-8) from the left Info Panel.

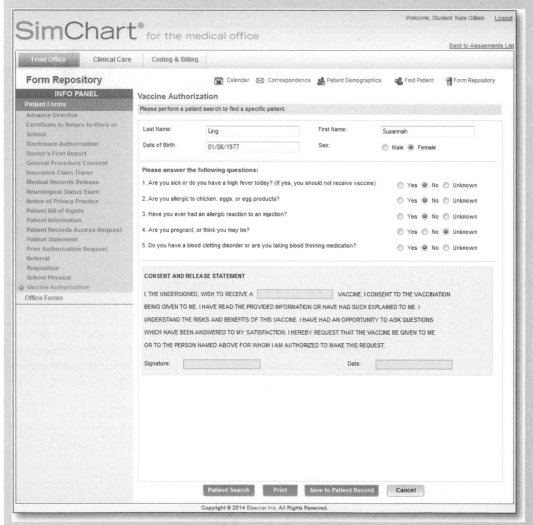

Figure 6-8 Vaccine Authorization.

2.   Click the Patient Search button to perform a patient search for Susannah Ling and confirm her date of birth. Some of Ms. Ling's information will auto-populate.

3.   Select the No radio button to indicate that Ms. Ling is not sick and does not have a fever.

4.   Select the No radio button to indicate that Ms. Ling is not allergic to chicken, eggs, or egg products.

5.   Select the No radio button to indicate that Ms. Ling has never had an allergic reaction to an injection.

6.   Select the Unknown radio button to indicate Ms. Ling's pregnancy status.

7. Select the No radio button to indicate that Ms. Ling does not have a blood clotting disorder and is not taking a blood thinning medication.

8. Click the Save to Patient Record button.

9. In order to print this form for Ms. Ling to sign, click the Find Patient icon to locate Ms. Ling's Patient Dashboard.

10. Scroll down to the Forms section within the Patient Dashboard and select the Vaccine Authorization.

11. Click the Print button to print the form in order to obtain Ms. Ling's signature.

EHR EXERCISE 6-9:   UPDATE IMMUNIZATION RECORD

Complete the following exercise in the EHR exercises environment of SCMO.

Document the following immunization that Dr. Martin ordered for Susannah Ling (01/02/1973): influenza, type TIV, dose 0.5 ml, administered IM in the right deltoid. Medical Corp. manufactures this immunization and the lot number is R5667. It expires 3 years from the current date. Ms. Ling does not have a reaction.

1. Within a patient encounter, select Immunizations from the Record drop-down menu.

2. Locate the Influenza (Flu) row and click on the green plus sign to the far right of that row. That row will become active so you can add an immunization to Ms. Ling's record.

3. Within the Type column, select TIV.

4. Within the Date Admin column, use the calendar picker to select the date administered.

5. Within the Provider column, type "Dr. Martin" in the text box.

6. Within the Route/Site column, type "IM/right deltoid" in the text box.

7. Within the Manufacturer/Lot# column, type "Medical Corp./R5667" in the text box.

8. Document the expiration date in the Exp column.

9. Within the Reaction column, type "No reaction" in the text box.

10. Click the Save button. A confirmation message will appear and the Immunizations table will display Ms. Ling's immunization.

Tracking Health Screenings and Immunizations

Health information often reaches patients in dribs and drabs. A woman may pick up a magazine at the hair salon and read about getting her daughter immunized against human papillomavirus (HPV), which causes certain types of cervical cancer. A man may hear about colon cancer screening from a colleague or neighbor who was not screened early and is now undergoing chemotherapy. A person with diabetes may be told by a friend with the condition that annual screening for diabetic retinal disease is necessary to detect vision-related complications of diabetes.

Unfortunately patients don't always get the advice they need from external sources. The information may be fragmented or just plain wrong. In addition, a patient's level of knowledge about healthcare often reflects disparities in income, education, age, and other variables. Tiro and colleagues studied a diverse group of American women to find out how much they knew about the role of HPV in causing cervical cancer. They found that those who knew the most were more likely to be younger, better educated, and more fully integrated into the healthcare system. The study did not measure income, but it's likely that those with better access to healthcare were in a higher tax bracket than those who did not visit a physician regularly.

In the past, relying on physicians to recommend appropriate screenings has been hit or miss. A general practitioner may be busy attending to the patient's chief concern—back pain or depression or bronchitis—or might not remember to order a screening test. Often the clinician isn't aware that the patient falls into a particular risk group.

That's where the EHR comes in. Clinical decision support tools take some of the burden off physicians and patients by showing the practitioner which conditions the patient is at risk for and flagging the patient's chart with appropriate screening reminders. However, it's still up to the provider to act on the reminder, and it's up to the patient to make and keep the screening appointment.

Of course, patients should also strive to be health literate (i.e., to stay as informed as possible about their health and to use this information to make well-considered health decisions). For example, they should learn the reason their physician is ordering a particular screening test. Depending on a patient's age and risk factors, certain testing should be done as part of a comprehensive health promotion plan. Children should be given the recommended immunizations, and adults should be vaccinated and screened for certain diseases, as indicated by their age, risk factors, or both (see Table 6-2). Screening tests might include mammograms, Pap tests, stool testing for occult blood, and laboratory tests such as a lipid (blood cholesterol) panel, complete blood count (CBC), and comprehensive metabolic panel (CMP). These tests either estimate a patient's risk for developing disease or detect its presence. A patient's insurance may or may not cover these kinds of screenings, so patients should check with their carrier before having them performed.

USING THE ELECTRONIC HEALTH RECORD FOR PATIENT EDUCATION

Healthcare providers can provide advice and treatment for the benefit of the patient. However, patients stand the best chance of living a healthy life by taking charge of their own health. The healthcare provider must create an atmosphere in which patients feel comfortable asking questions about their health status. Practitioners must also understand how to incorporate the resources they have within the office. These resources included written literature, videos or DVDs, educational group sessions, and even the EHR.

Although the main purpose of the EHR is to document patient-physician encounters, the EHR is also a useful tool for educating patients about their health and risk factors for disease. The EHR contains health data collected over a long time, allowing the attentive clinician to identify long-term trends that indicate elevated disease risk. For example, line graphs allow weight and blood pressure trends to be monitored and compared from visit to visit. Body mass index (BMI) is a simple but powerful health promotion tool the EHR provides (Trends and Applications 6-3).

TRENDS AND APPLICATIONS 6-3

Body Mass Index as a Health Promotion Tool

Inputting the weight and height into an EHR such as SCMO automatically calculates the patient's BMI. BMI is a height-weight ratio calculated by dividing the patient's weight (kg) by the square of his or her height (m²). The BMI is an inexpensive method of determining whether a patient is overweight or obese. It's a reliable indicator of body fatness because it has been shown to correlate strongly to the body fat percentage measured using highly accurate direct methods, such as underwater weighing. Scale weight measures pounds (or kilos, if you like)—but does not tell you whether a person is overweight.

TRENDS AND APPLICATIONS 6-3—cont'd

BMI is just a screening tool, though. As such, it indicates a risk for diseases related to overweight and obesity. However, taken by itself, a high BMI does not signal the presence of disease. The practitioner may choose to perform further tests or to counsel the patient about nutrition and physical activity. A person of normal weight generally has a BMI between 20 and 25. However, the mean BMI for an adult male in the United States is 26.6 and the average adult woman has a BMI of 26.5. Perhaps we wouldn't be wrong in suggesting that being an American has become a risk factor in itself.

EHR EXERCISE 6-10:   PREVENTATIVE SERVICES DOCUMENTATION

*Complete the following exercise in the EHR exercises environment of SCMO.

Susannah Ling (01/02/1973), shares her past preventative services with Dr. Martin during the patient interview. Within the past year she had a regular Pap smear on March 31, a general health panel lab test within normal limits on February 12, and an annual general eye examination within normal limits on June 24. Document these preventive services in Ms. Ling's record.

1. Within a patient encounter, select Preventative Services from the Record drop-down menu.

2. Click the Add button below the Procedures table.

3. Within the Add Procedure window, select Pap Smear from the Health Recommendation field.

4. Use the calendar picker to document the date in the Date Performed field.

5. Click the Save button.

6. Click the Add button below the Laboratory Testing table.

7. Within the Add Laboratory Testing window, select General Health Panel from the Health Recommendation field.

8. Use the calendar picker to document the date in the Date Performed field.

9. Click the Save button.

10. Click the Add button below the General Eye Exam table.

11. Within the Add General Eye Exam window, document "General eye exam" in the Health Recommendation field.

12. Use the calendar picker to document the date in the Date Performed field.

13. Click the Save button.

During an office visit patients are often given a great deal of information regarding their health status. It's helpful if patients have someone with them to help them understand and remember the details the healthcare staff provides. Written instructions help patients understand the disease process and learn to optimize quality of life while managing the symptoms of a chronic disease. The EHR stores patient information sheets on a broad range of topics that can be tailored for each patient and each visit.

As discussed in earlier chapters, the Internet is a great resource for accessing a broad range of health education and preventive medicine topics that can be tailored for each patient and every health issue. However, the medical office should establish a policy for distributing patient handouts generated from the Internet as well as a list of acceptable websites for the staff to use. Whether the education tool is maintained in the EHR system or outside on the web, the medical assistant should take time to review the printed materials with the patient. Proper communication skills are needed for the patient to fully understand the instructions. The following are a few guidelines for effective patient education:

- Speak with the patient in a quiet, well-lit area that offers as much privacy as possible.
- Take your time and don't rush as you explain the material.
- Provide both oral instructions and supplemental printed instructions from the EHR.
- Encourage the patient to ask questions as needed.
- Have the patient and caregiver demonstrate skills, such as insulin administration or wound dressing, before leaving the office to ensure that proper technique is used.
- Encourage patients to contact the office at any time with additional questions.

EHR EXERCISE 6-11:   PATIENT EDUCATION

*Complete the following exercise in the EHR exercises environment of SCMO.

Maria would like to learn more about her daughter Casey Hernandez's (10/08/2000) diagnosis of asthma. The medical assistant discusses asthma with Maria and prints a patient education handout for asthma. Document Person Taught as "Parent," and Printed Handout as Teaching Methods. During the patient education, Maria states the handout is very helpful to her understanding.

1. Within the Clinical Care module, perform a patient search to locate Casey Hernandez and confirm her date of birth.

2. Create an office visit for an established patient using the encounter options in the left Info Panel.

3. Select Patient Education from the Record drop-down menu.

4. Within the New tab, select Diagnosis from the Category drop-down menu.

5. Select Respiratory System from the Subcategory drop-down menu.

6. Select the Asthma check box in the Teaching Topics section. Use the View link to review the Patient Education handouts.

7. Select the Parent check box in the Persons Taught section.

8. Select the Printed Handout Given check box in the Teaching Methods section.

9. Select the No Barriers check box in the Learning Barriers section.

10. Select the Verbalizes Understanding check box in the Outcome section.

11. Click the Save button.

VITAL SIGNS

Every patient seen by the healthcare provider will have a set of vital signs—temperature, pulse, and respirations (TPR) and blood pressure (BP)—measured by the medical assistant. The record of these measurements must be documented in the EHR. Vital signs are an important part of the patient visit because they can indicate the presence of illness or disease. Extreme caution must be taken to ensure the accuracy of the measurements; thus they should be taken only by trained individuals.

Anthropometric measurements (from *anthropo-*, meaning "human"+ -*metry*, meaning "the process of measuring") are not considered vital signs but are generally obtained at the same time. These measurements include height (ht), weight (wt), BMI, and head circumference (in infants).

When the weight and height are recorded, many EHR systems automatically calculate the patient's current BMI. For blood pressure readings, you can also record the patient's body position (**postural BP**, or **posturals** (i.e., recumbent [reclining], sitting, or standing). During a well-child examination, the EHR can plot a child's height, weight, and head circumference on age-appropriate growth charts for percentile comparisons.

EHR EXERCISE 6-12:   ENTER VITAL SIGNS

*Complete the following exercise in the EHR exercises environment of SCMO.

The medical assistant measures the following vital signs for Casey Hernandez (10-08-2000) during today's office visit: Ht: 4 ft, 2 in; Wt: 82 lb; T: 99.2° F, forehead; P: 78, regular (radius); R: 16, regular; BP: 120.80, sitting, left arm with manual cuff; SpO_2: 99% (obtained with digital probe).

1. From the Simulation Playground, click on the Clinical Care Module.

2. Search and select patient record for Casey Hernandez (10/08/2000).

3. Enter the patient encounter (either select Existing Encounter from the Patient Dashboard, or create new encounter if no encounter exists).

4. Select "Vital Signs" from the Record drop-down box. The Vital Signs record is organized into a Vital Signs tab and a Height/Weight tab.

5. Within the Vital Signs tab, click Add button.

6. Document "99.2° F" as the temperature in the Fahrenheit field. Select Forehead from the Site drop-down menu. Notice the temperature is also displayed in Celsius after it is entered as Fahrenheit.

7. Document "78, regular" as the pulse and select Radial from the Site drop-down menu.

8. Document "16, regular" as the Respiration.

9. Document "120" as the systolic blood pressure and select Left arm from the Site drop-down menu. Document "80" as diastolic blood pressure and select Manual with cuff from the Mode drop-down menu. Select Sitting from the Position drop-down menu.

10. Document "99%" as the Oxygenation Saturation Percentage and select Digital probe, finger from the Site drop-down menu.

11. Click Save button.

12. Within the Height/Weight tab, click the Add button.

13. Document the height as "4 ft, 2 in" using the individual Height fields. Document the weight as "82" in the lb field. The BMI will auto-calculate.

14. Click the Save button.

ORDER ENTRY

One of the best ways to decrease the amount of errors and protect patients is being accomplished by adopting technology called computerized physician order entry (CPOE). The physician or other provider enters orders for the patient directly into the EHR, and the system automatically checks for safety and appropriateness. Besides the traditional medication orders, other procedures are maintained in the EHR system. Medical assistants, for example, will need to document the results of procedures performed in the office. For example, Snellen examination, glucometers, urinalysis, electrocardiograms (ECGs), and audiograms are all ordered and documented as part of the patient record.

EHR EXERCISE 6-13: IN-OFFICE ORDER ENTRY

*Complete the following exercise in the EHR exercises environment of SCMO.
Doctor Walden ordered a peak flow meter for Casey Hernandez (10-08-2000) (Figure 6-9). The Patient Goal was 490 and Casey tolerated the procedure without difficulty. During the three attempts, Casey obtained 450, 480, and 480.

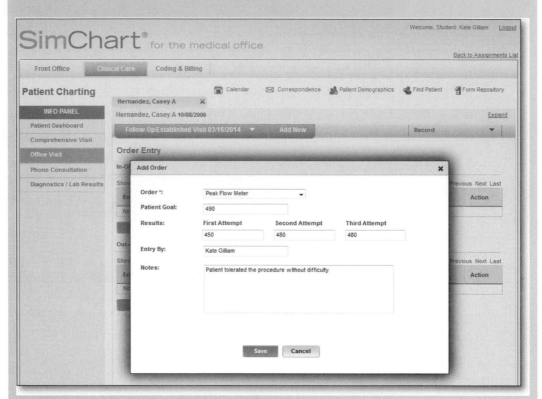

Figure 6-9 Peak Flow Meter; Add Order.

1. Within the Clinical Care module, perform a patient search to locate Casey Hernandez and confirm her date of birth.

2. Enter the encounter created during the previous exercise and select Order Entry from the Record drop-down menu.

3. Click the Add button located under the In-Office order grid.

4. Select Peak Flow Meter from the Order drop-down menu.

5. Document "490" in the Patient Goal field.

6. Document "450" in the First Attempt field.

7. Document "480" in the Second Attempt field.

8. Document "480" in the Third Attempt field.

9. Document your name in the Entry By field.

10. Document "Patient tolerated the procedure without difficulty" in the Notes field.

11. Click the Save button.

EHR EXERCISE 6-14:   OUT-OF-OFFICE ORDER ENTRY

*Complete the following exercise in the EHR exercises environment of SCMO.
  Dr. Walden would like to start Casey Hernandez (10-08-2000) on Accolate 20 mg twice daily for asthma management. Prepare a 3-month prescription with one refill and document this prescription in Casey's record.

1. Within the Clinical Care module, perform a patient search to locate Casey Hernandez and confirm her date of birth.

2. Enter the same encounter as the previous exercise and select Order Entry from the Record drop-down menu.

3. Click the Add button located under the Out-of-Office order grid.

4. Select Medication Prescription from the Order drop-down menu.

5. Select the check box for Julie Walden, MD.

6. Document "Asthma" in the Diagnosis field.

7. Document "Accolate" in the Drug field.

8. Select the Refill check box and document "1" in the Refill Details field.

9. Document "20 mg" in the Dose field.

10. Document "Tablet" in the Form field.

11. Document "By mouth" in the Route field.

12. Document "1" in the Refills field.

13. Document "Take 1 tablet po twice daily" in the Directions field.

14. Click the Save button.

15. Select Medications from the Record drop-down menu.

16. Within the Prescription Medications tab, click the Add button.

17. Within the Add Prescription window, select zafirlukast tablet (Accolate) from the Medication drop-down menu.

18. Select 20 from the Strength drop-down.

19. Select Tablet from the Form drop-down.

20. Select Oral from the Route drop-down.

21. Select 2 Times/Day from the Frequency drop-down.

22. Document "40 mg" in the Dose field.

23. Document "Asthma" in the Indication field.

24. Select the Active radio button to indicate the Status.

25. Click Save to view updated medication grid.

EHR EXERCISE 6-15:   RESPIRATORY ORDER REQUISITION

*Complete the following exercise in the EHR exercises environment of SCMO.
  Dr. Walden ordered Casey Hernandez (10-08-2000) to have spirometry (with and without inhalers) on December 23 for her asthma. The authorization number is TTY7800210. The test is ordered as routine. Remember to instruct Casey to bring her inhalers from home.

1. Click on the Form Repository icon.

2. Select Requisition from the left Info Panel.

3. Select Respiratory from the Requisition Type drop-down menu.

4. Click the Patient Search button to locate Casey Hernandez's record and confirm her date of birth.

5. Use the calendar picker to document December 23 of the current year as the Service Date.

6. Document "TTY7800210" as the Authorization Number.

7. Document "Julie Walden, MD" as the Ordering Physician.

8. Document the Diagnosis as "Asthma."

9. Document the Diagnosis Code as "J44.9."

10. Select the Spirometry (with and with inhalers) check box from the Respiratory Order section.

11. Select the Routine radio button to indicate that the examination is routine.

12. Document "Patient is to bring her inhalers from home with her" in the Patient Preparation field.

13. Click Save to the Patient Record.

THE PROGRESS NOTE

Progress notes are descriptions of the patient encounter. Accurately recording the details of a patient encounter ensures the highest level of patient care, decreases the risk of lawsuits, establishes evidence of illness, and documents the treatment plan. A patient note is created for every patient encounter. The most common method for organizing a patient encounter is called the *SOAPE note*. SOAPE is an acronym for the five components to be covered during a patient encounter: **s**ubjective data, **o**bjective data, **a**ssessment data, **p**lan of care, and **e**valuation. Let's look at each of these elements.

- **S: Subjective.** The **subjective** information is what the patient tells you. Generally, the problem is recorded in the patient's own words. For example, the patient might say, "Pain radiates down my left leg." Pain is a subjective (not observable or measurable to the clinician) symptom because, with present technology, we have no way to measure it other than the patient's self-report. It's akin to circumstantial evidence in a court of law—although the physician presumes the patient to be telling the truth, he or she would like some corroborating evidence before writing a script for Vicodin. That's where the "O" comes in.

- **O: Objective.** **Objective** information is that which can be observed, measured, or collected by the healthcare provider. Vital signs, anthropometric data, imaging studies, and laboratory tests are examples of objective data. Signs are objective, whereas symptoms are subjective. Objective data, in other words, are the forensic evidence of the medical chart—it is what it is. Interpretations may differ (as to what diagnosis it points to, for instance), but no one can argue with the data. A patient with leg pain, for instance, may have a measurable elevation of pulse and a measurable loss of reflexes, both of which would corroborate a report of pain.

- **A: Assessment.** The assessment is the practitioner's summation of the diagnosis or the impression of what's wrong with the patient. For example, after examining a pain patient, the assessment might be that he or she is suffering from sciatica, possibly caused by a herniated disk in the lumbar spine.

- **P: Plan.** The plan is just what it sounds like—the steps the provider plans to take to treat the patient. The physician may, for example, order an MRI of the lumbar spine to check for a herniated disk or may opt to order physical therapy.

- **E: Evaluation or Education.** The education section of the progress note is not always used by providers but when documented it includes advice to patients regarding treatments, advice to patients about disease, and future issues and response.

  Each physician has his or her own style of documentation. Some like to dictate paragraphs based on the history and examination of the patient, which results in the data being stored in an unstructured format. Others like to use a more structured method of documentation that enables easier medical research and formats the chart in an outline fashion. Physicians quickly rule out many things during their examination of a patient; the structured data method of documentation provides an easy way for them to document these rule-outs.

  Once the medical assistant has prepared the patient for the physician's examination or consultation, the physician sees the patient and documents the history, examination findings, plan of care, and any other observations made during the patient encounter. Physicians have choices for how they want to document in the medical record. The most efficient way is for the physician to carry a wireless tablet (like an iPad) or touch-screen laptop into the examination room with them. Some physicians are comfortable using a computer in front of patients, others are not. For physicians who are not comfortable keying documentation in front of patients, they can use a computer in the common hallway or in their office.

Digital Signature

Digitally signing a note is a great way to ensure a high level of security for a practice. When a note is signed electronically, the provider is representing that everything within the note is correct. A notation of when it was signed and by whom is shown below the signature line on the saved note. The digital signature process increases accountability and helps verify that the patient received the required care.

Although a batch of notes can be signed at once using the EHR, doing so may cause Medicare compliance problems. It's more prudent to sign the notes one by one as they are reviewed. The electronic signature is usually a password given to each provider. However, a note can be saved by selecting Cancel, and the provider can sign at a later time.

CHAPTER SUMMARY

- Proper documentation makes diagnosis and treatment more efficient, promotes patient safety, and provides evidence of the quality of care delivered for both legal protection and reimbursement purposes.
- Speech recognition is a technology that converts speech into text as the provider speaks into a microphone, eliminating the need for filing or transcription.
- An encounter allows the user to document all clinical documentation for the patient visit.
- The EHR is used to store and record documentation gathered from the patient interview, the review of systems, the patient history, chief complaint, vital signs, allergies, medication lists, and test results.
- The chief complaint (CC or cc) is the patient's main reason for seeking medical care. A patient may have more than one chief complaint. The history of the present illness (HPI) consists of a description of the patient's symptoms, their duration, a chronology of how the symptoms have changed, and an indication of what makes the problem better or worse.
- Allergies and medication use are important in the modification of patient treatment plans. Inaccurate documentation can lead to adverse reactions.
- Immunization history should be documented and monitored to ensure that a patient is up to date with necessary vaccinations. The immunization name, date, site given, route, person who administered, lot number, expiration, and manufacturer information should be documented in the EHR.
- A Problem List is a central location of the patient record where a summary of patient diagnosis can be referenced and is part of meaningful use reporting requirements.

- Patient education can support understanding and prevention of disease process and risk factors.
- Patient vital signs include temperature, pulse, respiration, and BP. Vital signs should be taken during every patient visit. The data collected are then entered into the EHR and can be pulled directly into the patient progress note.
- CPOE allows the user to document medical orders and reduce the incidence of medication errors.
- Progress notes are descriptions of the patient encounter and are the keystone of proper documentation. Accurately recording the details of a patient encounter ensures the highest level of patient care, decreases the risk of lawsuits, establishes evidence of medical necessity for treatment, and outlines the plan of care. The most common format for documenting a patient encounter is called the SOAPE method: **s**ubjective data, **o**bjective data, **a**ssessment, **p**lan, and **e**valuation.

CHAPTER REVIEW

Circle the Correct Term

Circle the term that correctly completes the sentence.

1. William comes to the office for the fourth time this year with bronchitis. This condition is **(acute, chronic)**.

2. Kimberly is complaining of an allergic reaction to an insect bite, a(n) **(acute, chronic)** condition.

3. Beverly reports having chickenpox when she was 11 years old. This is documented in the patient's past **(medical, family, social)** history.

4. Richard had a fracture of his right arm last summer. This is documented in the patient's past **(medical, family, social)** history.

5. Richie had called to make an appointment for a sore throat for 10 days. Upon questioning him, he also mentions difficulty swallowing and postnasal drainage. The patient's **chief complaint** is a **(sore throat, postnasal drainage, difficulty swallowing)**.

Key Terms Review

Match the term in column A to the definition in column B.

1. Subjective
2. Acute condition
3. E-visit
4. Chief complaint
5. Objective
6. Review of systems
7. Anthropometric measurements
8. High-alert medication
9. History of the present illness
10. Chronic condition
11. Medication reconciliation

a. An episodic illness or injury of limited duration that responds well to treatment

b. The process of comparing the medicatio list in the patient's EHR with the patient's self-report

c. An organized inventory of each organ system

d. Perceived only by the patient and not evident to or measurable by the clinician

e. Readily seen, perceived, or measured by the clinician

f. The height, weight, and size of the human body

g. A medication that poses a heightened risk of injury or death when improperly administered

h. A physician consultation with an established patient using a secure Internet service

i. A brief statement of the problem, condition, or symptoms that prompted the patient to seek medical care

j. The duration, location, severity, context, associated signs and symptoms, quality, and modifying factors related to a patient's illness

k. A prolonged illness that requires periodic follow-up

True/False

Indicate whether the statement is true or false.

1. _____Patient instructions should be performed in a well-lighted area with limited distractions.

2. _____Speech recognition software can distinguish one voice from another.

3. _____E-visits are illegal in most states.

4. _____Physicians using the EHR must use a structured method of data entry.

5. _____A medication reconciliation should be performed when a patient is removed from the operating room to the recovery room.

6. _____Voice recognition software does not eliminate the need to transcribe the provider's office notes.

7. _____The chief complaint includes all of the health concerns a patient is seen for during the course of a physician's visit.

8. _____The digital signature helps ensure the security of the patient's information.

9. _____Immunization status and administration need not be recorded for patients ages 18 and older.

10. _____A patient is asked for his or her allergy history only during the first visit.

11. _____A medication list must be reconciled and updated in the EHR during each patient encounter.

12. _____Many errors in EHR medication lists are attributable to patients' confusion about drug names and dosages.

Workplace Applications

Using the knowledge you obtained from the chapter, provide narrative answers to the following cases.

1. Document the following clinical data for Truong Tran (DOB: 05/30/1991). Create a patient encounter for today's Urgent Office visit.
   Chief Complaint: Pt. complains of right knee pain and swelling. Pain (4/10) started 3 weeks ago, after he fell while playing tennis. Patient states pain is sharp and constant. Patient has obtained some temporary relief by taking OTC medications.
   Allergies: Patient has no known allergies (NKA) to medications.
   Vital signs: Ht: 5′6″, Wt: 160 lb, T: 99° F, P: 66, R: 16, BP: 122/76 mg/dl

2. Al Neviaser (DOB 06/21/1968) has an appointment for a blood pressure check. Today his weight is 206 lb, his height is 67 in, and his blood pressure is 160/94 mm Hg sitting in the left arm. His pulse is 88 bpm regular. Use a follow-up visit encounter to document Mr. Neviaser's blood pressure check. Dr. Martin would like Mr. Neviaser to schedule a 30-minute appointment tomorrow at 2 PM to discuss his high blood pressure.

3. Paige is performing a patient interview. Determine whether the given data are part of the patient's personal (P), family (F), or social history (S).
   - Smokes one pack of cigarettes per day
   - Fixation of a broken right ankle in 1998
   - Tonsillectomy 25 years ago
   - Married with four children
   - Socially drinks alcohol, one or two servings per month
   - Mother died in 1990 of breast cancer
   - Grandfather diagnosed with colon cancer

4. Casey Hernandez (DOB 10/08/2000) is recovering from the flu and needs a note to excuse her from school. She was absent Monday and Tuesday of this week. Use the Form Repository to generate an excuse from school for Casey.

5. Update the Casey Hernandez (10/08/2000) problem list to include asthma.

6. Susannah Ling is ordered a glucometer. Her random blood sugar (RBS) at 10 AM is 110 mg/dl. Document these results in In-Office Order Entry.

7. During Al Neviaser's visit, the physician requests a patient education handout for hypertension. The medical assistant prints and reviews the handout with the patient. He verbalizes understanding, and no learning barriers are present.

BIBLIOGRAPHY

Baxter, S., Farrell, K., Brown, C., et al. (2008). Where have all the copy letters gone? A review of current practice in professional-patient correspondence. *Patient Education Counseling*, 71, 259–264.

Committee on Identifying and Preventing Medication Errors. (2006). In: P. Aspden, J. Wolcott, & J. L. Bootman, Eds. *Preventing medication errors: Quality chasm series.* National Academies Press: Washington, DC. Available at: www.nap.edu/openbook.php?recordid=11623&;page=R1. Accessed 11.06.11.

Heubusch, K. (2008, August). Physician practices and information management. *Journal of American Health Information Management Association*, 79, 18–22.

Katz, H. P., Kaltsounis, D., Halloran, L., et al. (2008). Patient safety and telephone medicine: Some lessons from closed claim case review. *Journal of General Internal Medicine*, 23(5), 517–522.

Krishna, Y., & Damato, B. E. (2005). Patient attitudes to receiving copies of outpatient clinic letters from the ocular oncologist to the referring ophthalmologist and GP. *Eye (London, England)*, 19, 1200–1204.

Mangin, W. (2008). Tapping HIM expertise for physician practice EHRs. *Journal of American Health Information Management Association*, 79(10), 8.

Medicare Learning Network. (2008). *Evaluation and management services guide.* Centers for Medicare & Medicaid Services: July. Available at: http://fsmaonline.org/MEDICARE%20E&M%20GUIDE.pdf. Accessed 11.06.11.

Mendelson, R. A. (2008). Dot your i's and cross your t's: Tips on avoiding indefensible medical records. *American Academy of Psychiatry News*, 29(6), 19, 29.

National City. (2007). *Going paperless: Do electronic health records hold value for your practice?* Cleveland, Ohio: National City Corporation. Available at: www.summahealthnetwork.org/media/12421/12476.pdf. Accessed 11.06.11.

Orrico, K. B. (2008). Sources and types of discrepancies between electronic medical records and actual outpatient medication use. *Journal of Managed Care Pharmacy*, 14(7), 626–631.

Rouf, E., Chumley, H. S., & Dobbie, A. E. (2008). Electronic health records in outpatient clinics: Perspectives of third year medical students. *BMC Medical Education*, 8, 13.

Schmitt, B. D. (2008). Telephone triage liability: Protecting your patients and your practice from harm. *Advances in Pediatrics*, 55, 29–42.

Soto, C. M., Kleinman, K. P., & Simon, S. R. (2002). Quality and correlates of medical record documentation in the ambulatory care setting. *BMC Health Services Research*, 2(1), 22.

The Joint Commission. (2008). *Sentinel event alert: Preventing pediatric medication errors.* Available at: www.jointcommission.org/SentinelEvents/SentinelEventAlert/sea_39.htm. Accessed 16.02.09.

Tiro J. A., Meissner H. I., Kobrin S., Chollette V. (2007). What do women in the U.S. know about human papillomavirus and cervical cancer? *Cancer Epidemiology Biomarkers Prevention*. 16:288–294.

U.S. Department of Health and Human Services. (2003). Healthy weight, overweight, and obesity among U.S. adults. *National Health and Nutrition Examination Survey.* Available at: www.cdc.gov/nchs/data/nhanes/databriefs/adultweight.pdf. Accessed 20.3.14.

Wick, J. Y. (2007). Reducing risk through medication reconciliation. *Pharmacy Times.* Available at: www.pharmacytimes.com/issues/articles/2007-03_4438.asp. Accessed 14.02.09.

Young, A., & Proctor, D. (2007). *Kinn's the medical assistant: An applied learning approach* (10th ed.). St Louis: Mosby.

chapter 7

Using the Electronic Health Record for Reimbursement

Chapter Outline

Commission on Accreditation of Allied Health Education Programs (CAAHEP) Competencies

1. Discuss principles of using electronic medical records (EMRs).
2. Execute data management using electronic health records such as the EMR.
3. Perform procedural coding.
4. Perform diagnostic coding.
5. Compare processes for filing insurance claims both manually and electronically.

Chapter Objectives

1. Discuss the role of the patient, the provider, and the third-party payer in the medical reimbursement process.
2. Define medical coding.
3. Discuss diagnostic coding classifications, and outline the CPT-4 coding system.
4. Evaluate the advantages and disadvantages of the pay-for-performance (P4P) incentive model.
5. List the information contained in a typical Superbill, and explain how the form is used in an outpatient facility.
6. Post charges, payments, and adjustments to a patient ledger.

7. Discuss the concept of medical necessity, and indicate how it affects third-party reimbursement.

8. Complete HIPAA 5010 compliant claims.

9. Complete a Day Sheet.

10. Define fraud and abuse, explain the difference between the two, and give examples of each.

Key Terms

abuse   Unintentional deception in which a provider inappropriately bills for services that are not medically necessary, do not meet current standards of care, or are not medically sound.

coding variance   Medical coding mistakes caused by computer error or by various kinds of human error, from simple carelessness to incorrect application of coding guidelines and procedures.

compliance plan   A written set of office policies and procedures intended to ensure compliance with laws regulating billing, coding, and third-party reimbursement.

CPT-4 (Current Procedural Terminology, fourth edition)   A comprehensive set of medical codes and corresponding labels that describes procedures, treatments, and services for the purpose of determining reimbursement rates.

electronic data interchange (EDI)   An information exchange technology that facilitates the rapid, accurate transfer of encrypted data in a standardized, mutually agreed-upon format.

encounter form   A form generated to reflect the services and charges for a patient visit. It includes patient information, account balance, and follow-up instructions.

fraud   Presenting (or causing to be presented) claims for services that an individual or entity knows or should know to be false.

guarantor   The person who bears ultimate financial responsibility for a patient's account; usually the guarantor is the patient, but the guarantor for a minor or a person of decreased mental capacity may be a parent, trustee, or legal guardian.

HIPAA 5010   The standard claim format used by a noninstitutional provider or supplier to submit a claim electronically to Medicare and most other insurance carriers for covered services.

ICD-10-CM   International Classification of Diseases, Tenth Revision, with Clinical Modification. A coding system used to describe inpatient and outpatient diagnoses.

medical coding   The process of assigning standard numeric or alphanumeric codes to diagnoses, procedures, and treatments for research, disease tracking, and reimbursement purposes.

medical identity theft   The unauthorized use of someone else's personal information to obtain medical services or submit fraudulent medical insurance claims for reimbursement.

pay for performance (P4P)   An outcomes-based payment model that offers providers financial incentives for meeting specific standards and electronically documenting compliance with them; punitive measures may be applied to providers who fail to comply.

HEALTHCARE REIMBURSEMENT

For many providers and staff, submitting insurance claims is a tedious task. But the implementation of electronic health records (EHRs) and interoperable practice management systems has made it much easier. At first, learning the reimbursement requirements for several insurance payers can seem overwhelming, but it's more useful to think of billing and coding activities as a kind of puzzle—perhaps one of those brain teasers in which you compare two drawings side by side and try to spot subtle differences between them. Or maybe handling practice finances is more like deciphering a word-find puzzle, requiring attention to detail and complex pattern-recognition skills. To solve it, categorization and memory skills, inductive logic, and persistence are needed. Of course, having experience and using a bit of strategy can be helpful, too. Working with medical reimbursement means submitting claims to big insurance companies or to the federal government (Medicare or Medicaid), who are known as third-party payers. Who, then, are the first and second parties? The patient or **guarantor,** and provider, respectively. Most healthcare plans require that patients pay for a portion of their care. Cost sharing might include both copayment and coinsurance. One way to keep the medical office outstanding balance from creeping up is to require the patient to pay a copayment at the time the service is rendered.

Fortunately, having an EHR makes billing functions a snap compared with a traditional billing system. It's like the difference between preparing your own tax return with paper and pencil and using tax preparation software to accomplish the task. Most EHR systems, including SimChart for the Medical Office (SCMO), have integrated practice management systems. Patient accounts are handled with practice management software, which creates a patient statement for provider services rendered. This statement serves as a patient receipt and provides documentation for insurance claim processing.

The Health Insurance Portability and Accountability Act **(HIPAA) 5010** is an electronic claim format used to gather reimbursement from Medicare and most other insurance payers. Electronic claims are not printed out and are transmitted via a modem. This method of **electronic data interchange (EDI)** saves money and is quicker than mailing handwritten claim forms. Electronic submission also decreases the amount of errors on the claim submission and provides a faster reimbursement. In addition, HIPAA requires that all claims be submitted electronically for all covered entities. The law does make some exceptions for small physicians' offices.

REVENUE CYCLE

The Healthcare Financial Management Association (HFMA) defines revenue cycle as "[a]ll administrative and clinical functions that contribute to the capture, management, and collection of patient service revenue." In other words, revenue cycle management starts with the scheduling of a patient and continues through the collection of the last payment for services rendered.

When the front office person schedules a new patient for an appointment to see the physician, he or she will gather some preliminary information about who will be paying the bill. When patients arrive for their appointment, the front office person will scan patients' picture identification cards and insurance cards to allow the billing department access to this information. This is the start of the revenue cycle. Correct identification of the patient and the patient's payers including the appropriate payer numbers will be the difference between a paid or denied claim. Patients' medical insurance information frequently changes. The medical staff must verify a patient's eligibility every time the patient comes into the office.

In the previous chapter you learned that the clinical documentation serves as the basis for charges that appear on the bill. Timely (preferably at the point of care) and accurate capture of the clinical documentation is therefore the next step in the revenue cycle.

When the patient is ready to leave the healthcare facility, it is important to collect any monies due. This revenue cycle step starts the exchange of money. The patient will be asked to pay for any copayment amount due; in the case of self-pay patients, they will be asked to pay for all of the services rendered.

EHR EXERCISE 7-1: ADD A PATIENT SECONDARY INSURANCE PLAN

*Complete the following exercise in the EHR exercises environment of SCMO.

Celia Tapia (05/18/1970) now has secondary medical insurance coverage effective 06/24/2014. The new payer is MetLife. The policy holder is Arnold Tapia (SSN 812-93-1341). Policy ID number is YYT1230990, group number is TR508. Claims are submitted to 1234 Insurance Avenue, Anytown, AL 12345. The claims phone number is 800-123-4444.

1. Click the Patient Demographics icon.

2. Use the patient search fields to locate Celia Tapia's record. Click the blue "Celia" hyperlink displayed in the List of Patients table to view Ms. Tapia's demographics.

3. Within the Patient Demographics window, click the Insurance Tab to add the secondary insurance carrier.

4. Select MetLife from the drop-down menu in the Insurance field.

5. Document "Arnold Tapia" in the Name of the Policy Holder field.

6. Document "812-93-1341" in the SSN of the Policy Holder field.

7. Document "YYT1230990" in the Policy/ID Number field.

8. Document "TR508" in the Group Number field.

9. Document "1234 Insurance Avenue" in the Claims Address 1 field.

10. Document "Anytown" in the City field.

11. Select AL from the State drop-down menu.

12. Document "12345" in the ZIP field.

13. Document "800-123-4444" in the Claims Phone field.

14. Click the Save Patient button.

CODING SYSTEMS

To standardize the way claims are submitted, whether on paper or electronically, diagnostic and procedural coding systems are used. **Medical coding** is the process of assigning standard numeric or alphanumeric codes to diagnoses, procedures, and treatments for reimbursement purposes. Code determination is based on medical documentation in the patient chart or record, which serves as evidence of patient care. In addition, researchers use coding systems as a means of gathering data to monitor trends in the incidence of acute and chronic illnesses, infectious diseases, injuries, and poisoning.

Proper code assignment is not an exact science because even a single code can reflect many variables, all of which are ultimately related to the complexity of the patient's condition and thus the amount of time, attention, and expertise required to treat the person.

The most common coding systems used in the medical office are the following:

1. Diagnosis codes: International Classification of Diseases, 10th revision, with Clinical Modification (ICD-10-CM). Implementation date is tentatively set for October 2015.

2. Procedure codes: Current Procedural Terminology, 4th edition (CPT-4)

Role of the Electronic Health Record in Medical Coding

The EHR stores complete sets of codes and links them to the appropriate coding labels gathered from the patient progress note. Coding systems are updated annually; therefore, the codes must be updated annually in the EHR as well. It's important for the medical coder to double-check the codes assigned by the software. Computers *do* make mistakes. Moreover, a qualified health information technology (HIT) specialist can address faulty assignment of codes, at least in part, by tweaking certain administrative options and defaults within the program. But first the problem must be recognized.

Billing and collections processes are done most often by practice management software, which is often integrated into an EHR like SCMO. Once the practice has received a payment, the payment must be posted to the correct patient's account. Part of the medical assistant's job is to ensure that patients are billed and credited properly, to see that insurance claims are submitted correctly, and to follow up on unpaid claims and delinquent patient accounts.

CRITICAL THINKING EXERCISE 7-1

What other skills do you think would contribute to the ability to code swiftly yet accurately?

CRITICAL THINKING EXERCISE 7-3

Why do you think the amount of time spent with the patient does not weigh as heavily as the other three factors in determining the proper E/M code?

An EHR can determine the proper E/M code based on the provider's documentation. A prompt will be generated if more information is required to select the right code. The EHR might, for example, ask the user to check off more morbidity and mortality risk factors from a list, or to specify which questions the patient was asked during the history taking. The system factors in other data, too, such as how long the visit lasted, the type of visit (office visit vs. consultation), and the kind of patient (new vs. established). Then the program crunches the data to generate the appropriate code. This saves the coder time by eliminating the need to manually generate a specific procedure code; however, the job responsibility now is to make sure the codes are up to date and correct for what the physician performed.

Many EHR systems allow you to see the impact of your coding choices before committing to them. Of course, the actual documentation made by the provider during a visit should not be altered by anyone except the provider. In many cases, however, two virtually identical labels are available to *describe* that documentation. Ordinarily, CMS regulations allow you to choose the one that is more favorable to practice revenues.

If you like the changes you've tested and believe they accurately reflect the level of service provided during the patient's visit, you may save them. If you think a different set of codes would give you a more favorable outcome, you can scrap your changes and try a different coding scheme or return to the original CPT code (Trends and Applications 7-2). When in doubt, check with the provider because all reimbursement requests may be subject to audits by the payer.

TRENDS AND APPLICATIONS 7-2

Pumping Up Practice Revenues

"God does the healing," Benjamin Franklin once quipped, "and the physician takes the fee." We might like to think practice revenues are of no concern to us, but maintaining financial records and overseeing medical billing are two important aspects of the medical assistant's administrative scope of practice, as defined by the American Association of Medical Assistants.

Besides, fattening the physicians' wallets has its perks, starting with job security. If the providers who own the practice believe you're looking after their financial interests and caring for their patients, you'll quickly become indispensable to them. In addition, a thriving practice is less likely to lay off staff.

Then, of course, there's the matter of raises, which tend to be commensurate with each staff member's value to the practice. You might even consider becoming a certified coder. Many providers are willing to help their medical assistants pay for such credentialing as a means of retaining qualified medical assistants. Having dual certification in medical assisting and coding is a surefire way to boost your own reimbursement! If you decide to change jobs down the road, you'll be able to show potential new employers how the billing and coding practices you implemented increased practice revenues. The list below is a good place to begin.

When a claim is denied, check the simplest explanation first. Most claims are kicked back to the physician because of transposed digits, incorrect modifiers, and other elementary errors. Double-check and resubmit denied claims.

Learn as much as you can about diseases and their treatment, including common procedures. According to the American Health Information Management Association (AHIMA), lack of knowledge in these areas is at the root of many coding variances, especially with the implementation of ICD-10-CM coding.

TRENDS AND APPLICATIONS 7-2—cont'd

Take advantage of government resources, such as the Medicare Coverage Decisions website, for Medicare coding updates.

Use the coding features of your EHR to test several codes before deciding which to use. As long as your codes are accurate, CMS rules allow you to select the more profitable of two similar code selections.

Take advantage of the reporting capabilities of the EHR to track denied claims by provider and by billing code. This will help you identify trouble spots so you can work with the providers and other staff members to find targeted solutions.

Treat coding and reimbursement training as a continuous process rather than as a one-time cram session. Use the EHR's messaging capabilities to circulate information about coding modifications, newly issued codes, and coding tips.

Don't neglect to bill for your own time. The practice can bill for medical assisting services during an established patient's office visit lasting about 5 minutes for which the presence or supervision of a physician is not required (see CPT code 99211 for details). Use the EHR to track trends in the number of medical assisting visits billed.

Anesthesia (00100-01999). This section is used to report the administration of anesthetic usually during surgery by an anesthesiologist, anesthetist, or other physician. Anesthesia means introducing a drug to obtain partial or complete loss of sensation in a patient. The codes used include local, regional, and general anesthesia.

Surgery (10021-69990). The surgery section makes up the bulk of the CPT manual. It categorizes surgical procedures by body system, such as the integumentary (skin), respiratory, musculoskeletal, cardiac, and reproductive systems. These codes are used to report a variety of surgical procedures performed in medical offices and in outpatient surgical centers, and to code inpatient surgeries.

Radiology (70010-79999). Radiology is the study of using radiant energy to diagnose and treat patient conditions. Codes listed in the radiology section describe radiologic imaging services, including diagnostic and therapeutic radiology, nuclear medicine, ultrasound, computed tomography, and magnetic resonance imaging.

Pathology and Laboratory (80048-89399). Pathology and laboratory codes are used to describe providers' orders for blood panel tests, such as complete blood counts, and for blood tests to check for conditions such as anemia (low blood iron content), hyperglycemia (high glucose content, which could indicate diabetes), and coagulation disorders.

Diagnostic immunology tests, which check the blood for the presence of antigens and antibodies to specific substances, fall within this category as well. Tests for conditions as diverse as pregnancy, rheumatoid arthritis, illegal drug use, and exposure to HIV are all classified as immunologic tests. Even the typing and crossmatching of blood that's done before major surgery falls into this area.

Pathology and laboratory codes are also used for anatomic pathology procedures, such as Pap tests (cell pathology) and microscopic examination of tissue specimens (surgical pathology). For example, excised moles, intestinal polyps, or biopsied lung tissue may be examined microscopically for evidence of malignancy.

Medicine (90281-99607). The medicine section of the Category I CPT-4 code manual includes tests, procedures, and other services not covered in other sections of the CPT manual. These services for coding diagnostic and therapeutic services are considered to be fairly noninvasive. Examples include injections and immunizations, allergy testing, psychiatry, ophthalmology, and neurology services.

Category I Guidelines. A set of guidelines is given at the beginning of each section of the CPT-4 Category I manual. Reading them will save you time in the long run, even if the information doesn't make for fascinating conversation at the next office picnic. The guidelines clarify terms, list procedures found within the section, and suggest codes to use for unlisted procedures. Two-digit numeric modifiers are often added to the CPT codes to specify more precisely which procedure was performed. A full list of modifiers and their descriptions is provided in Appendix A of the CPT-4 manual.

Category II

Category II codes are supplemental codes used to help researchers collect data, track illness and disease, and measure quality of care. The use of these codes is not required, and there is no reimbursement value attached to using them.

Category III

Category III codes are temporary codes applied to emerging technology. These codes are used to minimize the number of unlisted codes being submitted to report services not otherwise described in Category I codes.

CRITICAL THINKING EXERCISE 7-4

Do you think every member of the medical office staff, including providers, should have to attend mandatory training on coding topics, or just those who code? Explain your answer.

ICD-9-CM Coding

The ICD-9-CM coding system translates complex medical diagnoses and procedures into a universal language used by healthcare providers to request reimbursement for inpatient hospital services and hospital-based outpatient services and doctor office visits. The system is overseen by CMS and the National Center for Health Statistics.

Like any language, both sides—payers and providers—understand it. Once the healthcare provider assesses, consults with, examines, or treats the patient and documents the encounter in a progress note, a diagnosis code is assigned or generated automatically by the EHR. It's important to remember that the code must directly reflect the doctor documentation, without making assumptions. If there is any question, the healthcare provider should be consulted.

The ICD-9-CM code book consists of three volumes:

- **Volume 1: Tabular List of Diseases.** This section lists diseases in numeric order by code number. It contains 17 chapters for classifying diseases by etiology (cause) or anatomic site. In addition, it includes a list of V codes and E codes. V codes describe factors that influence a patient's health status and contact with health services. These codes are used when a patient is seen for a wellness examination and even to further describe the circumstance under which a patient was ill. E codes detail external causes of disease, injury, and poisoning. These codes are optional for use and are never used as the primary code for a patient claim. The duty of the E code is primarily to provide details about an accident or patient injury and to help to identify whether the patient visit is related to automobile or employment. Examples of V codes and E codes:
  - Julian and Robert are celebrating the birth of their daughter Elizah in the hospital. This birth of a single live baby in the hospital would be coded as a V30.0.
  - Noah is allergic to penicillin. This affects the way he is treated for infections and is documented in his medical record. The V code for "history of allergy to penicillin" is V14.0.
  - Travis accidentally fell out of bed. This E code would be documented as E884.2.
  - An E997.1 would be used to report an injury due to biological warfare.
- **Volume 2: Alphabetic Index of Diseases.** This volume contains diagnostic terms that do not appear in Volume 1. It's used as a guide to help locate the complete code in Volume 1.
- **Volume 3: Tabular List and Alphabetic Index of Procedures.** The third volume of the ICD-9-CM code is used by hospitals. These codes are used to report inpatient care and are not intended for use by ambulatory care practices.

ICD-10-CM Coding

When you decide to take on a career in healthcare, it is important to remember that the field is always changing. It's an exciting time in healthcare with the implementation of EHRs, healthcare reform, and **ICD-10-CM.** Up until now, the United States has been the only country not using ICD-10-CM and still using a legacy system, ICD-9. The ICD-10-CM coding system has been delayed several times, and current legislation passed on April 2, 2014 doesn't nail down a definitive switch date from ICD 9, despite a mention of October 2015. Table 7-1 outlines the basic differences between ICD-10-CM and ICD-9-CM coding systems. There are several reasons for the transition from ICD-9-CM to ICD-10-CM:

Table 7-1   Differences Between ICD-10-CM and ICD-9-CM Coding Systems

ICD-9-CM	ICD-10-CM
3-5 characters	3-7 characters
First character is numeric or alpha (E or V)	First character is alpha
Characters 2-5 are numeric	Characters 2-7 are alpha or numeric
Always at least 3 characters	Always at least 3 characters
Use of decimal after 3 characters	Use of decimal after 3 characters

1. ICD-9-CM codes do not accurately reflect the current procedures and technology being performed.
2. The healthcare industry cannot accurately measure quality of care using ICD-9-CM codes due to the lack of specificity. ICD-10-CM codes will allow for a more detailed classification of the patient's condition or injury.
3. Improved efficiencies and lower costs
4. Reduced coding errors
5. Alignment of the United States with coding systems worldwide

Like any language, both sides—payers and providers—understand it. Once the healthcare provider assesses, consults with, examines, or treats the patient and documents the encounter in a progress note, a diagnosis code is entered by the user or generated automatically by the EHR. It's important to remember that the code must directly reflect the physician documentation, without making assumptions. If there is any question, the healthcare provider should be consulted.

The ICD-10-CM code book consists of about 70,000 codes and the system has these characteristics:

- Three to seven alphanumeric characters. The first character is a letter. The second and third characters are numbers (for example: J44.9, Bronchitis with airway obstruction).
- ICD-10 has 21 chapters without supplementary classifications.
- Coding conventions are the same as ICD-9, with the addition of a placeholder "x," use of seventh character, Excludes Notes, Code Also note, and default codes and syndromes.

Like the ICD-9-CM manual, the ICD-10-CM code sets are organized into the following:

Tabular List of Diseases. The Tabular List is organized by chapters based on body systems, conditions, and etiology; signs and symptoms; injuries and poisonings; factors influencing health status; and external causes of morbidity. The codes are listed in numeric or alphanumeric order. A set of coding notes appears at the beginning of each chapter, or subdivision of each chapter.

Alphabetic Index of Diseases. This volume contains diagnostic terms to guide the location of a complete code. It contains an alphabetic index of disease and injury, Table of Neoplasms, and Table of Drugs and Chemicals.

Official Guidelines for Coding and Reporting. The Guidlines are divided into four sections.

Learning new systems, or any system for that matter, can seem overwhelming. But as with anything, practice and attention to detail will make all the difference. Just remember all of us in healthcare are going through the same transition, and together it can be a success for both the practice and the patient.

EHR EXERCISE 7-2: DOCUMENT ICD-10-CM IN THE PROBLEM LIST

*Complete the following exercise in the EHR exercises environment of SCMO.

Kyle Reeves (01/01/1996) is here for his follow-up appointment with Julie Walden, MD, for irritable bowel syndrome. He was first diagnosed with this problem on January 21 of this year. Update the Problem List using ICD-10-CM.

1. Click the tab for the Clinical Care module.

2. Perform a patient search for Kyle Reeves and confirm his date of birth.

3. Enter the existing encounter (if no encounter is available, create a follow-up encounter using the workflow described in Chapter 6).

4. Select Problem List from the Record drop-down menu.

5. Click the Add Problem button.

6. In the Add Problem window, select Irritable bowel syndrome from the Diagnosis drop-down menu.

7. Select the ICD-10 Code radio button and document "K58.9" as the diagnosis code. Refer to ICD-10-CM to confirm.

8. Using the calendar picker, document the Date Identified as 01/21 of this year.

9. Select the Active radio button.

10. Click the Save button.

PAY FOR PERFORMANCE

Pay for performance (P4P) is an outcomes-based payment model that rewards providers for delivering evidence-based care according to specific standards and for electronically documenting compliance with those standards. This model is quickly becoming the gold standard by which most health plans (such as health maintenance organizations [HMOs] and preferred provider organizations [PPOs]) operate. These "bonus" structured payments systems are quickly turning into earned revenue as providers strive to meet specific patient targets or measures. For this reason, these value-based systems are shifting away from fee-for-service systems into a combination of fee-based and performance-based payment systems.

Incentives and Penalties

To ensure that practices participate in P4P programs, private insurers and Medicare have built disincentives into the system for those who fail to meet P4P standards. For example, in 2009, providers who used a computerized physician order entry (CPOE) system to submit claims for Part D Medicare recipients were rewarded with performance pay amounting to 2% of their annual Medicare billing. This bonus has slowly been phased out, and by late 2014, it will no longer be offered. Providers who choose not to use CPOE will be dinged with a penalty equal to 1% of their annual Medicare billing, increasing incrementally to 2% in 2015 and thereafter. The AMA has spoken out against this and other policies that reduce reimbursement based on substandard results.

CRITICAL THINKING EXERCISE 7-5

Do you believe P4P programs work to improve patient care? What other factors might motivate practitioners to improve patient care?

Use of the Electronic Health Record in P4P Compliance

Because P4P is an outcomes-based model, technology is required to measure and document the outcomes achieved. That's where the EHR system comes in. The EHR offers a way to record improvement by noting laboratory results, findings of imaging studies, and clinical progress notes. Providers who haven't adopted an EHR are at a distinct disadvantage in adhering to the program's requirements. Because hospitals and other large institutions were the first to implement electronic records systems, the P4P model has been widely used in those settings. However, large practice groups, multi-physician practices, and even solo practitioners are now being asked or even required to participate in P4P programs. The P4P model works best when applied to patients with chronic illnesses, such as diabetes, hypertension, and arthritis. Most of these patients are treated by primary care providers in solo or small group practices of five or fewer physicians. Such practices treat nearly 70% of all ambulatory care patients in the United States.

Contrary to the stereotype of the wealthy physician, these providers often have middle-class incomes and operate their practices on shoestring budgets. They may not have the financial wherewithal to purchase an EHR and to endure a prolonged period of reduced productivity during the transition from a paper office to a wired one. Medical assistants need to understand how the system works because it affects not just reimbursement, but also how patient care is delivered in order to achieve the outcomes specified by the program.

SUPERBILL

Practice management systems attach a Superbill (also known as an *encounter form, walkout form, route slip, fee slip,* or *checkout form*) to the patient's visit for use during an office visit. In a paper-based office this form is typically printed in triplicate: one copy for the insurance reimbursement specialist to reference during claim preparation, one copy for the patient, and one copy for the office. This form is used by the medical biller to create a claim for reimbursement of services.

Patient demographics and insurance information change frequently, so patient information must be verified at the beginning of every visit. Both sides of the insurance card should be scanned and updated right away if the policy has changed. It's also important to remember that codes change annually. The Superbill must be updated to reflect any coding changes.

The patient's copy of the **encounter form** serves as a bill and evidence of care. This form documents charges for the office visit, any past due amounts, and a record of payment by the patient. The final copy is used by the office to audit claims and chart documentation.

Of course, using an EHR vastly simplifies the process of completing a Superbill. In SCMO, the Superbill can be completed by using the Progress Note Fee Schedule for reference. This clinical record describes the services performed during the patient visit. The Superbill serves as a summary of visit events and can help with the tracking of diagnosis codes or procedure usage. The purpose of the Superbill is twofold: to collect data about the patient and to record details of the patient's visit. The form includes the following information:

- Demographic data (patient's name, address, phone number, and date of birth)
- Date of appointment
- Guarantor (the person responsible for the account)
- Insurance policy number and group ID
- Problem and diagnosis codes
- Service codes and ranking
- Account balance

EHR EXERCISE 7-3: SUPERBILL

*Complete the following exercise in the EHR exercises environment of SCMO.

Complete the Superbill for Kyle Reeves (01/01/1996) for a problem-focused, established patient visit performed today for irritable bowel syndrome. (Be sure you created the encounter from EHR Application 7-1 first.) The patient has a $10.00 copayment for office visits. Kyle's mother Kim has paid the copayment in cash.

1. Click the tab for the Coding and Billing module.

2. Select Superbill from the left Info Panel.

3. Perform a patient search for Kyle Reeves and confirm his date of birth.

4. Select the correct encounter in the Encounters Not Coded table (Figure 7-1).

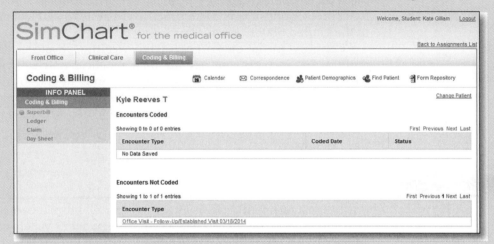

Figure 7-1 Encounters Not Coded.

5. Within the first step of the Superbill, document "$10.00" in the Copay field (Figure 7-2).

6. Document "$0.00" in the Previous Balance field.

7. Click the Fee Schedule link in the top right corner to determine the charges for the office visit and document "$32.00" in the Today's Charges field.

8. Document "$10.00" in the Today's Payment field.

9. Document "$22.00" in the Balance Due field.

10. According to Kyle's Patient Demographics, he is covered by Kim Reeves. Document "Kim Reeves" in the Insured's Name field.

11. Click the Same Address as Patient.

12. Select the Child radio button for the Patient Relationship to Insured field.

13. Select the Single radio button for the Patient Status field.

14. Select the No radio button to indicate that there is no other health benefit plan.

15. Select the No radio buttons to indicate that the patient condition is not related to employment, an auto accident, or other accident.

16. Click the Save button.

17. Click the Next button.

18. Select the ICD-10 radio button.

19. Document "Irritable bowel syndrome, K58.9" as the first diagnosis in the Diagnosis box.

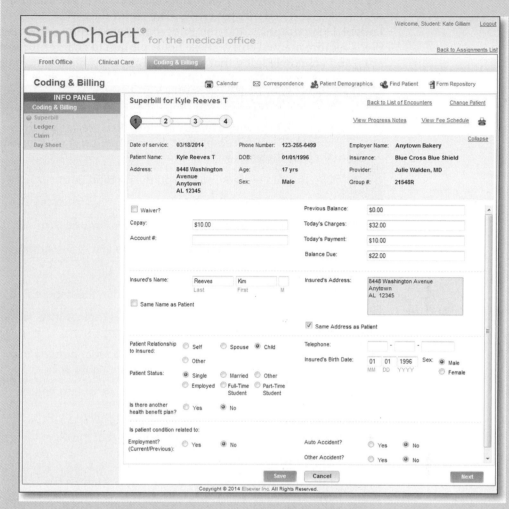

Figure 7-2   Superbill, page 1.

20. Document "1" in the Rank column for Problem focused in the Office Visit box, followed by "32.00" in the Fee column and "99212" in the Est column. Click the Fee Schedule link in the top right corner for reference.

21. Click the Save button.

22. Because this was the only service provided, click the Next button twice to progress to the fourth page of the Superbill.

23. Scroll to the bottom of the fourth page of the Superbill and select the check box to indicate that you are ready to submit the Superbill.

24. Select the Yes radio button to indicate that a signature is on file.

25. Enter today's date in the Date field.

26. Click Save button.

27. Click the Submit Superbill button.

HIPAA 5010 CLAIM PROCESSING

Once the Superbill is submitted, it's time to request reimbursement of services from the third-party payers. The electronic format of the claim form is HIPAA 5010. This form lists the patient information: name, address, insurance, diagnosis codes, services, charges, along with the provider and payment information for the payer to review. Once the claim is submitted, it is paid, pending, or denied. It is important for the medical assistant to accurately complete and review the claims prior to submission to decrease the incidence of denials due to data entry errors. The claim data in SCMO is pulled from two sources: Patient Demographics and the Superbill. Aside from the auto-populated fields, several fields require manual entry. These fields pertain to charges for services, assignment of benefits, and acknowledging that a HIPAA form is on file for the patient.

EHR EXERCISE 7-4:　PREPARE A CLAIM

*Complete the following exercise in the EHR exercises environment of SCMO.

　　Using the Superbill completed in EHR Application 7-2 for reference, prepare a Claim for Kyle Reeves's visit.

1. Click the tab for the Coding and Billing module.

2. Select Claim from the left Info Panel.

3. Perform a patient search for Kyle Reeves and confirm his date of birth.

4. The submitted Superbill appears in the List of Superbills for Kyle Reeves.

5. Click the Superbill to progress to the Claim.

6. Review the information auto-populated in the Patient, Provider, and Payer tabs.

7. Within the Encounter tab, select the Yes radio button to indicate the HIPAA form is on file, and document the date.

8. Within the Claim Info tab, select the No radio buttons to indicate that Kyle's condition is not related to employment or an auto accident.

9. Select the Yes radio button in the Release of Info field.

10. Select the Yes radio button in the Assignment field.

11. Select the Yes radio button to indicate that the signature is on file.

12. Click the Save button.

13. Click the Charge Capture tab.

14. Document "03/18/2014" in the DOS From and DOS To columns.

15. Document "99212" in the CPT/HCPCS column.

16. Document "1" in the POS column. Click the Place of Service link in the top right corner for reference.

17. Document "32.00" in the Charge column. This amount will auto-populate in the Total Charges field below the table.

18. Document "10.00" in the Amount Paid 10.00 field below the table. The $22.00 the patient owes will auto-populate in the Balance Due field.

19. Click the Save button.

20. Click the Submission tab.

21. Select the check box to indicate that you are ready to submit the Claim.

22. Select the Yes radio button to indicate that Kyle's signature is on file.

23. Document the date in the Date field.

24. Click the Save button.

25. Click the Submit Claim button to submit the Claim electronically.

26. In order to print your work to turn in to your instructor, select the correct encounter within the table to reenter a read-only view of the claim you submitted electronically. Click the printer icon in the top right corner. The work completed within the claim will display as a PDF in a separate window. (NOTE: The print functionality within the 5010 is only to submit your 5010 form to your instructor or save in a portfolio. This does *not* generate a 1500 form).

MEDICAL NECESSITY

Medical necessity is a legal doctrine that holds that medical services rendered must be reasonable and necessary according to generally accepted clinical standards. Claims that fail to meet such standards will be denied. Furthermore, if claims deemed medically unnecessary are discovered during an audit, Medicare or the insurance carrier may demand that the provider pay back the reimbursement received for such services. A pattern of such claims may indicate intentional fraud, in which case the practitioner would be likely to lose his or her Medicare provider eligibility, have his or her medical license revoked, and endure criminal prosecution.

The provider's establishment of medical necessity ensures that a patient's treatment is consistent with the diagnosis and is provided in the appropriate setting under adequate supervision. Clinical decision support (CDS) systems can significantly aid providers with selecting treatments that are consistent with the diagnosis. SCMO and other EHR systems automatically line up the most likely orders for the chief complaint, thus enabling the physician to place orders based on necessity. By monitoring procedures and testing, insurance payers can ensure that the correct level of care is being provided.

If the clinician believes a service might not be covered, preauthorization to perform the procedure should be obtained before scheduling it. Preauthorization may be done over the phone, by fax, or electronically. Regardless of the method, the patient's insurance information, diagnosis, service requested, and clinical information must be provided. It's also smart to ask the patient to agree in writing to pay for the procedure if the claim is denied.

A little planning goes a long way when you're requesting a preauthorization. Make sure you have all the information you need at hand before making the call. Once it has been approved, the authorization number and expiration date should be documented in the EHR. The procedure can then be scheduled. Remember that every insurance contract has its own set of guidelines regarding which services and procedures require authorization. Creation of an insurance manual can help you keep track of these requirements. In addition, the EHR's reporting capabilities can be used to identify codes that are being consistently rejected.

EHR EXERCISE 7-5: DOCUMENTING A PRIOR AUTHORIZATION REQUEST

*Complete the following exercise in the EHR exercises environment of SCMO.

Dr. Walden ordered physical therapy for Erma Willis (12/09/1947) three times a week beginning today and lasting for the next 2 weeks for degenerative disk disease of the lumbar spine. The order is effective starting today and expires in 30 days. The service will be performed at Eagle Physical Therapy located at 0301 Gunner Way in Anytown, AL 54622. This order is not related to an injury or workers' compensation. The authorization number is GUN02282013.

Use the Form Repository of the Simulation Playground to complete this Prior Authorization Request.

1. Click Form Repository icon in the top right corner.

2. Select Prior Authorization Request from the left Info Panel.

3. Click the Patient Search button to locate Erma Willis and confirm her date of birth.

4. Document "Julie Walden, MD" in the Ordering Physician field.

5. Document your name in the Provider Contact Name field.

6. Document "Eagle Physical Therapy located at 0301 Gunner Way, Anytown, AL 54622" in the Place of Service field.

7. Document "Physical Therapy" in the Service Requested field.

8. Document the date in the Starting Service Date field.

9. Document 2 weeks from the current date in the Ending Service Date field.

10. Document "3 times a week for 2 weeks" in the Frequency field.

11. Document "DDD M51.3" in the Diagnosis/ICD Code field.

12. Select the No radio buttons to indicate that this request is not injury related or workers' compensation related.

13. Document "GUN02282013" in the Authorization Number field.

14. Document the date in the Effective Date field.

15. Document the expiration date of 30 days in the Expiration Date field.

16. Click the Save to Patient Record button.

17. Access the Forms section of the Patient Dashboard to print the form if required.

PATIENT LEDGER

There is much more to maintaining a patient in the EHR than just clinical documentation. The billing information is also stored in a central location inside the EHR. A summary of all payments, charges, and adjustments to a billing account in SCMO is called the Ledger. The Ledger is organized by guarantor, but the search for the account is still performed using the patient's name (Figure 7-3). Proper entry of the guarantor in the Patient Demographics screen will facilitate the creation of the correct ledger in the Coding and Billing module. The Ledger, located in the left Info Panel of the Coding and Billing module is not linked to a patient encounter, which allows the user to document payments and charges at any time. At the end of the day, the medical assistant documents all payments and charges processed during the day on the Day Sheet, which acts as a summary of accounting for a specific date. The information documented within the Day Sheet is then used to complete a Bank Deposit Slip, located in the Office Forms section of the Form Repository.

Figure 7-3
Ledger search.

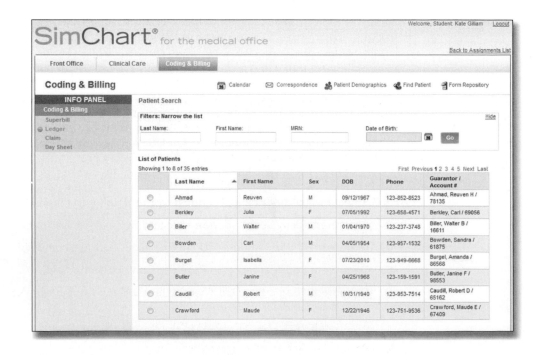

EHR EXERCISE 7-6:   PATIENT LEDGER

*Complete the following exercise in the EHR exercises environment of SCMO.
    Document the copayment and charge for Kyle Reeves's (01/01/1996) office visit billed today in the Account Ledger of the Coding and Billing module.

1. Click the tab for the Coding and Billing module.

2. Select Ledger from the left Info Panel.

3. Perform a patient search for Kyle Reeves and confirm his date of birth.

4. The Ledger for Kyle Reeves will display "Ledger for Guarantor: Kim Reeves" because she is Kyle's mother and is responsible for his account.

5. Document the date in the Date column using the calendar picker.

6. Document "Kyle Reeves" in the Patient column.

7. Document "99212" in the Service column.

8. Document "32.00" in the Charges column.

9. Document "10.00" in the Payment column.

10. Document "0.00" in the Adjustment column. The Balance of $22.00 is auto-popu-lated based on the amounts listed in the previous columns (Figure 7-4).

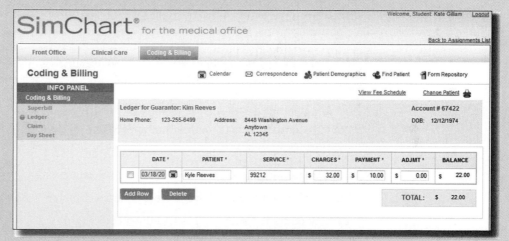

Figure 7-4   Ledger title.

11. Click the Save button.

EHR EXERCISE 7-7:   DAY SHEET

*Complete the following exercise in the EHR exercises environment of SCMO.
    Document the daily transactions on a Day Sheet using the payments listed be-low. Use the Fee Schedule in SCMO to determine the correct service code and fee. No adjustments were made during any of these transactions. Once all transactions are documented, complete the Daily Posting Proof, Accounts Receivable, and Deposit Proof sections of the Day Sheet.

- Mora Siever (01/24/1964) paid $10.00 for an expanded problem-focused office visit. Her account did not have a balance prior to today's visit.
- Erma Willis (12/09/1947) paid $20.00 for an anoscopy. Her account had a balance of $140.15 prior to today's visit.
- Celia Tapia (05/18/1970) paid $0.00 for a spirometry. Her account had a balance of $58.00 prior to today's visit.

1. Click the tab for the Coding and Billing module.

2. Select Day Sheet from the left Info Panel.

3. In the first row, document the date using the calendar picker.

4. Document "Mora Siever" in the Patient Name column.

5. Document "99213" in the Service column.

6. Document "43.00" in the Charges column.

7. Document "10.00" in the Payment column.

8. Document "0.00" in the Adjustment and Old Balance columns.

9. Document "33.00" in the New Balance column.

10. Click the Add Row button.

11. In the second row, document the date using the calendar picker.

12. Document "Erma Willis" in the Patient Name column.

13. Document "46600" in the Service column.

14. Document "64.00" in the Charges column.

15. Document "20.00" in the Payment column.

16. Document "0.00" in the Adjustment column

17. Document "184.15" in the New Balance column.

18. Document "140.15" in the Old Balance column.

19. Click the Add Row button.

20. In the third row, document the date using the calendar picker.

21. Document "Celia Tapia" in the Patient Name column.

22. Document "94010" in the Service column.

23. Document "78.00" in the Charges column.

24. Document "0.00" in the Payment column.

25. Document "0.00" in the Adjustment column

26. Document "136.00" in the New Balance column.

27. Document "58.00" in the Old Balance column.

28. Within the Daily Posting Proof section, document the total for Column E (198.15) + Column A (185.00) = Subtotal (383.15) – Column B (30.00) = Subtotal (353.15) – Column C (0.00) = Column D (353.15)

29. Within the Accounts Receivable Proof section, beginning with the total Accounts Receivable Previous Day (2300.00) + Column A (185.00) = Subtotal (2485.00) – Column B (30.00) = Subtotal (2455.00) – Column C (0.00) = Accts Receivable for Day (2455.00).

30. Document "30.00" in the Deposit Proof section.

31. Click the Save button.

32. Access saved Day Sheets by clicking the Saved Day Sheets tab and selecting the correct date from the drop-down menu (Figure 7-5).

Continued

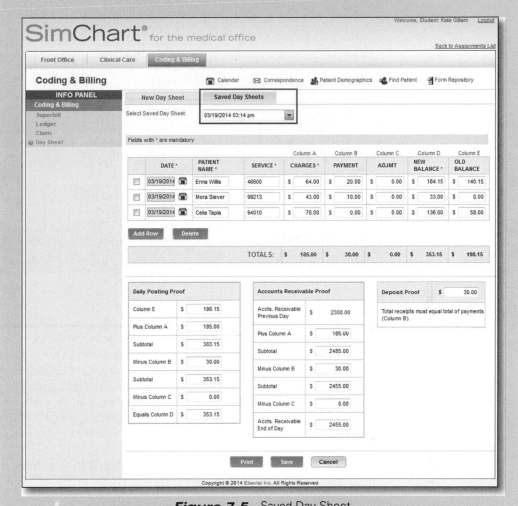

Figure 7-5   Saved Day Sheet.

CRITICAL THINKING EXERCISE 7-6

Which other functions of the EHR can help to streamline billing and coding practices? How would you integrate them into the office routine?

EHR EXERCISE 7-8:   CREATE AN INSURANCE CLAIM TRACER

*Complete the following exercise in the EHR exercises environment of SCMO.

While reviewing claims, the medical assistant notices an outstanding claim for Mora Siever (01/24/1964) for an ECG with interpretation for mitral valve prolapse (MVP) on 07/08/2011. The claim number is 1357246 and it was submitted to Aetna on 07/09/2011. The service fee is $89.00.

1. Click Form Repository icon in the top right corner.

2. Select Insurance Claim Tracer from the left Info Panel.

3. Click the Patient Search button to locate Mora Siever and confirm her date of birth.

4. Document "1357246" in the Claim # field.

5. Document "Aetna" in the Billed To field.

6. Document your name in the Contact Person field.

7. Document "84066" in the Account Number field.

8. Document "Self" in the Insured field.

9. Document "07/09/2011" in the Date of Claim field.

10. Within the table, document "07/08/2011" in the Date(s) of Service column.

11. Document "93000" in the Procedure column.

12. Document "I34.1" in the Diagnosis field.

13. Document "07/09/2011" in the Date Billed field.

14. Document "89.00" in the Amount field.

15. Document "89.00" in the Total field below the table.

16. Click the Save to Patient Record button.

FRAUD AND ABUSE

Fraud is misrepresentation of the medical services provided to deceive or mislead another person or entity, such as Medicare. Fraudulent schemes are carried out primarily for financial gain. Sometimes physical or emotional harm is inflicted on patients or others in the process. Regardless of the motive, fraud is unacceptable and is not tolerated by the government, by private insurers, or by patients. They may be able to fly under the radar for a time, but once exposed, few courts have any sympathy for those who cheat the system. Judges don't hesitate to impose stiff fines and to see to it that these swindlers spend some time in orange jumpsuits.

Medical identity theft is a different kind of fraud in which the patient—or someone posing as one—is the con artist. The victim is a current patient or any person who has healthcare coverage.

CRITICAL THINKING EXERCISE 7-7

The federal government is cracking down on bogus companies set up for the sole purpose of shaking down taxpayers for millions of dollars in Medicare funds. Search the web on this topic. What other examples of Medicare fraud can you find?

✔ SECURITY CHECKPOINT 7-1

Medical Identity Theft

Medical identity theft is a particular kind of fraud that occurs when a criminal steals personally identifying details about a patient, such as a health insurance identification number or Social Security number, and uses the information either to pose as the patient to obtain healthcare services or to submit false insurance claims (such as claims for Medicare benefits) for reimbursement. In rare cases, a criminal may perpetrate a medical identity theft for another reason, such as to avoid being prosecuted for using illicit drugs or for obtaining prescription drugs illegally.

This crime harms its victims in two ways: medically and financially. The medical harm comes from having the victim's medical record riddled with false information that can be traced to the imposter's medical history. That means a patient's medical history and EHR can include someone else's information. In some cases the entire file can contain the wrong patient's medical history. This erroneous information can be life threatening, such as when the real patient has a drug allergy and the imposter doesn't, or when the patient and the imposter have different blood types.

The damage can create financial disarray that takes years to sort out. Unpaid medical bills may lead to a dismal credit score. The imposter may have expensive hospitalizations, surgeries, and other treatments that push the real policy owner above the insurer's lifetime caps. Extensive claims may make it impossible for the victim to purchase new medical insurance.

To make matters worse, victims may not be aware that a theft has occurred until years later, when they develop a medical condition or are tracked down by creditors seeking payment for bills racked up by the imposter. The thief seeking care or fraudulent reimbursement under someone else's name often arranges to have bills and other correspondence sent to a post office box to avoid alerting the real policy owner of the fraud. This allows the scammer to conceal the crime for a long time.

Unscrupulous office workers and employees of healthcare systems are paid as much as $15 for palming off the medical information of a single patient. That's a princely sum compared with the chump change a waiter pockets—as little as 40 cents—for swiping a diner's credit card information and selling it online. Although the interoperability of EHR systems may make it easier for thieves to steal entire databases of patient information, most security consultants agree that an electronic file is infinitely more secure than any mailbox.

Abuse is an unintentional deception in which a provider inappropriately bills for services that are not medically necessary, do not meet current standards of care, or are not medically sound. The difference between fraud and abuse is this: fraud occurs when a provider bills for services that were never rendered or were not rendered at the level of service indicated, whereas abuse takes place when dubious or excessive tests and treatments are administered.

Once the abusive practice has been recognized, efforts must be made to retrain the employee so the abusive practice is stopped. If a healthcare worker is suspected of performing fraudulent practices, it must be reported to a supervisor immediately. You, as a healthcare professional and patient advocate, have a responsibility to your patient and your employer. Examples of fraud and abuse are given in Box 7-1. The best way to ensure that your office is not engaging in abusive practices is to create and enforce a compliance plan.

BOX 7-1
Examples of Fraud and Abuse

Fraud
Falsifying a physician's note
Altering test results
Misrepresenting the person who provided the service in order to bill at a higher level
Falsifying dates of service
Inserting codes for services not documented in the patient progress note
Submitting duplicate claims for reimbursement
Changing the diagnosis to receive a higher level of reimbursement, a practice known as "upcoding"
Offering patients kickbacks, gifts, or perks of any kind to accept services that can be billed to Medicare
Failing to refund credit balances due to patients or third-party payers
Balance billing (billing the patient for the difference between the provider's fee and the Medicare allowable amount)
Abuse
Calling patients back for repeated and unnecessary visits
Charging excessively for services and supplies
Performing more diagnostic tests than necessary
Using different fee schedules for Medicare recipients and those with private insurance
Waiving fees and deductibles

CHAPTER SUMMARY

- In the medical reimbursement process, claims are submitted by the provider (the second party) to Medicare or a private insurance carrier (the third-party payer) on behalf of the patient (the first party). It's within the medical assistant's scope of practice to ensure that patients are billed and credited properly, to see that insurance claims are submitted correctly, and to follow up on unpaid claims and delinquent patient accounts.

- Medical coding systems are used in the physician's office as a standardized way of submitting diagnostic and procedural information from a patient encounter. Codes are used primarily for reimbursement purposes, but they're also useful to researchers in collecting data.

- The ICD-9-CM and ICD-10-CM coding system translates complex medical diagnoses into a uniform language used to facilitate reimbursement and tracking of diagnoses. CPT-4 codes are used to report services and procedures performed by the healthcare provider.

- The P4P payment model rewards providers for delivering evidence-based care according to specific standards and for electronically documenting compliance with those standards.

- The Superbill is attached to every patient visit, and the physician uses it to record the procedure and diagnosis codes for the visit. In addition, the encounter form details patient demographics, insurance information, charges, payments, and any balance due.

- The concept of medical necessity holds that services rendered must be reasonable and necessary according to generally accepted clinical standards.

- Fraud is misrepresentation of the medical services provided to deceive or mislead, usually for the purpose of financial gain. Abuse occurs when a provider defrauds Medicare or insurance companies by rendering services that are inappropriate or not medically necessary.

CHAPTER REVIEW ACTIVITIES

Fill in the Blanks

Read the scenario and fill in the blanks.

Janelle uses the _____ filled out by the physician during the office visit to submit claims. The form includes procedure codes from the _____ coding manual and diagnostic codes from the _____ coding manual to complete the _____ for submission to the insurance company. Once the claim has been submitted, the _____ reviews the claim and provides reimbursement for the patient visit.

Key Terms Review

Match the term in column A to the definition in column B.

1. HIPAA 5010
2. ICD-10-CM
3. Third-party payer
4. CPT-4
5. Electronic data interchange (EDI)
6. Compliance plan
7. Encounter form
8. Guarantor
9. Fraud
10. Pay for performance (P4P)
11. Coding variance
12. Copayment
13. Medical identity theft
14. Medical coding
15. Abuse

a. Presenting (or causing to be presented) claims for medical services that an individual or entity knows or should know to be false

b. The party financially responsible for the patient's healthcare services

c. Assigning standard numeric or alphanumeric codes to diagnoses, procedures, and treatments for reimbursement purposes

d. The person who bears ultimate financial responsibility for a patient's account

e. An outcomes-based payment model that offers providers financial incentives for meeting specific standards

f. A document given to the patient during each visit that lists the diagnosis and procedure codes most often used in the practice, along with other pertinent information

g. A coding system used to describe hospital-based outpatient services and physician office visits

h. The unauthorized use of someone else's personal information to obtain medical services or submit fraudulent medical insurance claims for reimbursement

i. Technology that makes possible the rapid, accurate transfer of encrypted data in a standardized format

j. Medical codes and labels that describe procedures, treatments, and services for the purpose of determining reimbursement rates

k. Standard claim format used by a noninstitutional provider or supplier to bill Medicare and most other insurance carriers for covered services

l. Unintentional deception in which a provider inappropriately bills for services that are not medically necessary, do not meet current standards of care, or are not medically sound

m. A written set of office policies and procedures intended to ensure compliance with laws regulating reimbursement

n. Medical coding mistakes

o. A fixed, out-of-pocket expense for covered services

True/False

Indicate whether the statement is true or false.

1. _____ The HIPAA 5010 claim format cannot be filed electronically.

2. _____ Code assignment is ultimately related to the complexity of the patient's condition and thus the amount of time, attention, and expertise required to treat the person.

3. _____ Coding systems are updated annually with new, revised, and deleted codes.

4. _____ The medical assistant is permitted to correct minor errors in physician documentation.

5. _____ CPT codes were revised using actual clinical cases as models to draft codes appropriate for use in general practice and in a multitude of specialty areas.

6. _____ Evaluation and management codes are used to describe office visits for new and established patients.

7. _____ The P4P payment model has forced many providers to return to paper-based record keeping.

8. _____ The encounter form allows patients to rate physician performance and post coded ratings on an Internet site.

9. _____ Encounter forms are not used by offices implementing an EHR. The EHR directly links the patient visit with the corresponding charges.

10. _____ Medical necessity ensures that the appropriate diagnosis is linked to the proper procedure.

Matching

Link the appropriate diagnosis with its procedure.

1. DJD of the lumbar spine
2. Heart disease
3. Asthma
4. Abdominal pain
5. Dizziness
6. Hyperlipidemia

a. KUB
b. Pulmonary function test (PFT)
c. Stress test
d. MRI of lower back
e. CT of brain
f. Lipid panel

Workplace Applications

1. Daniel Miller (03/21/2012) is in the office for left ear pain. His father states he has been pulling at his ear for the past 3 days and is not sleeping through the night, but denies any fever or runny nose. Daniel has no known allergies and is not on any medications. His vital signs are Wt: 28 lb, T: 97.9° F taken on the forehead, R: 20, and P: 112, regular. Dr. Martin determines that Daniel's lungs are clear to auscultation. The examination on the neck is supple with no lymphadenopathy noted, and there are no other significant findings. Dr. Martin determines a diagnosis of otitis media. The plan of care is over-the-counter pain medications and antihistamines, and Dr. Martin instructs Daniel's father to bring him back to Walden-Martin in 1 week if his condition does not improve. Create an urgent care visit for Daniel and document the following information in the Progress Notes.

   S: C/O left ear pain. Father states child is pulling at his ear for the past 3 days and is not sleeping through the night. Denies fever or runny nose. NKA. Not taking any current medications.

O: Vital signs: Weight 28 lb, T: 97.9° F (forehead), Pulse: 112, regular, R: 20. LUNGS: Clear to auscultation. NECK: Supple, no lymphadenopathy. No significant finding

A: otitis media

P: OTC pain medications and antihistamines. RTC 1 week if not better.

2. Complete the Superbill and Ledger for Daniel Miller's (03/21/2012) established problem-focused visit today.

3. Create a claim for Daniel Miller's visit today.

4. Dr. Able has asked you to be in charge of a new compliance team for the prevention of fraud and abuse practices. What types of employees would you ask to be part of the team? The agenda of the first meeting will be to define fraud and abuse and provide examples of each. Once you have compiled a list, discuss solutions and proper ways to handle these situations. Define for your team the penalties for fraudulent activities.

5. Complete the Bank Deposit Slip for today. The following money is on hand:

Currency:	$210.00	
Coin:	$2.25	
Checks	$10.00	#455
	$45.00	#321
	$20.00	#1051

EHR in Review

1. Dr. Martin's patient, Daniel Miller (3-21-2012), presents for an appointment today. He is being seen for a wellness examination. The physician ordered a MMR vaccine, which the medical assistant administered. Create a Wellness encounter and document the MMR in the immunization record.
Immunization: MMR 0.5 ml given to the left (IM) vastus lateralis. The manufacturer is Hospira Lab and the lot number is 4578T. The expiration date is 01/16/2020. No reaction is noted.

2. Complete a Superbill for Daniel Miller's MMR injection. There is no copay for the service. Use the Fee Schedule to obtain the fees for both the MMR and administration fee.

3. Update the Ledger for Daniel's injection today.

4. Complete a Claim for Daniel's service today.

5. Results of a radiology examination ordered by Jean Burke, NP, came in today for Tai Yan (04/07/1956). Use the Diagnostics/Lab Results tab in the left Info Panel of the Patient Dashboard to document the results of the lumbar spine x-ray performed last Tuesday: Impression; Moderate Degenerative Disk Disease.

BIBLIOGRAPHY

Adams, W. L. (2009). *Coding and reimbursement: A simplified approach* (3rd ed.). Philadelphia: Saunders.

American Association of Medical Assistants. (2007–2008). *Occupational analysis of the CMA (AAMA).* Available at: http://aama-ntl.org/medassisting/OA.aspx. Accessed 03.02.09.

American College of Emergency Physicians. *Documentation, compliance plan keys to avoiding fraud and abuse allegations.* Available at: www.acep.org/practres.aspx?id=30314. Accessed 05.02.09.

Denny, S. (2008). Queuing up for quality: Boosting quality with electronic work queues. *Journal of American Health Information Management Association, 79*(1), 32–36.

e-HIM Work Group on Benchmark Standards for Clinical Coding Performance Measurement quality subgroup. (2008). Collecting root cause to improve coding quality measurement. *Journal of American Health Information Management Association, 79*(3), 71–75.

Fitzgerald, F. (2007). The pitfalls of pay for performance. *Journal of the National Medical Association, 99*(2), 123–124.

Fordney, M. (2007). *Medical insurance handbook for the physician's office* (10th ed.). Philadelphia: Saunders.

Glendinning, D. (2008). E-prescribers see Medicare bonus, but late adopters will face pay cut. *American Medical News*, Aug 4. American Medical Association. Available at: www.ama-assn.org/amednews/2008/08/04/gvl10804.htm. Accessed 02.02.09.

Hoover, E. L. (2007). "Payment for performance" will be good for the medical profession and patients. *Journal of the National Medical Association*, 99(2), 125–127.

Krier-Morrow, D. (2007). 10 practical tips for pulmonary practices. American Thoracic Society. Available at: www.thoracic.org/sections/career-development/practitioners-page/practice-tips/articles/tip29.html. Accessed 03.02.09.

Leibenluft, J. (2008). Credit card numbers for sale: How much does a Visa or MasterCard number go for these days?. *Slate*, Apr 24.

Locke, R. G., & Srinivasan, M. (2008). Attitudes toward pay-for-performance initiatives among primary care osteopathic physicians in small group practices. *The Journal of the American Osteopathic Association*, 108, 1. Available at: www.jaoa.org/cgi/content/full/108/1/21#REF12. Accessed 02.02.09.

Miller, N. W. (2002). What is medical necessity?. *Physicians News Digest*, Aug. Available at: www.physiciansnews.com/law/802.miller.html. Accessed 05.02.09.

National Center for Health Statistics. (2006). *Health, United States, 2006*. (Vol. 384). U.S. Department of Health and Human Services, Hyattsville, MD. Available at: www.cdc.gov/nchs/data/hus/hus06.pdf#117. Accessed 02.02.09.

O'Reilly, K. B. (2008). P4P found to have little impact on care quality. *American Medical News*, Aug 4.

Paduda, J. (2008). PacifiCare fined $3.5 million for claims-processing violations. *Healthcare Economist*, Jan 31. Available at: http://healthcare-economist.com/2008/01/31/pacificare-fined-35-million-for-claims-processing-violations. Accessed 31.03.14.

Taché, S., & Chapman, S. (2005). What a medical assistant can do for your practice. *AAFP's Family Practice Management*, 12(4), 51–54. Available at: www.aafp.org/fpm/20050400/51what.html. Accessed 31.03.14.

chapter 8

The Personal Health Record

Chapter Outline

Commission on Accreditation of Allied Health Education Programs (CAAHEP) Competencies

1. Recognize the role of patient advocacy in the practice of medical assisting.
2. Advocate on behalf of patients.
3. Identify types of records common to the healthcare setting.
4. Use the Internet to access information related to the medical office.

Chapter Objectives

1. Define and explain the purpose of keeping a personal health record (PHR).
2. Describe the three ways of storing PHR data, and outline the advantages and drawbacks of each.
3. Describe how a PHR can be synchronized with medical devices, such as blood pressure cuffs, blood glucose meters for patients with diabetes, and peak flow meters for patients with asthma.
4. Discuss the need for interoperability between PHR systems, electronic health records (EHRs) systems, and related systems.
5. Explain how direct-to-consumer laboratory services can help protect a patient's privacy.
6. Discuss the benefits for consumers and for providers of creating a PHR.
7. Identify steps in setting up a PHR.
8. Identify steps in maintaining the PHR.

Key Terms

advance directive   A binding legal document prepared and signed by a competent individual outlining the person's wishes should the person become incapacitated. Components of an advance directive may include a medical power of attorney and a living will.

caregiver   A person responsible for providing physical care and emotional support, usually in a home-care setting, to a person who is ill, disabled, or dependent.

host   A server that provides data transfer, storage space, and other services to users at remote locations; a host has a unique domain name and is, in effect, the point at which a website originates.

living will   The part of an advance directive that specifies which life-sustaining treatments (for example, mechanical ventilation and tube feeding) should be administered or withheld if the person becomes incapacitated.

medical power of attorney (also called durable power of attorney for healthcare or healthcare proxy)   The part of an advance directive naming a trusted person to make medical decisions on the patient's behalf should he or she become unable to make such decisions independently.

online community   A virtual meeting space where like-minded people with common interests or concerns interact and build relationships using real-time chat rooms, asynchronous threaded discussions, discussion groups, social media, news groups, web conferencing, and other technologies.

patient-controlled health record   The portion of a patient portal that contains data loaded by the patient and to which he or she alone may grant or deny access.

patient portal   A website that serves as an information transfer hub between patient and physician and provides information and services, such as secure email, search capabilities, access to an online appointment book, and limited access to patient records.

personal health record (PHR)   A secure, comprehensive record of health information that is controlled by the individual, creating a confidential electronic or paper-based file that is easy to access, manage, and share.

populate   To complete a template or create a record by filling in a set of predetermined fields with information ranging from demographic data to values and measurements (for example, vital signs) to entire documents (such as correspondence and operative reports).

social networking   The practice of using online communities to expand one's social or business contacts and exchange content, such as images and instant messages; the term also refers to the broader phenomenon of this practice, which has created virtual communities with millions of members.

Wi-Fi (short for Wireless Fidelity, a technologic certification body)   A means of connecting wirelessly to the Internet using a local area network or router.

WHAT IS A PERSONAL HEALTH RECORD?

In the old days we had personal hygiene, personal checks, and personal pronouns. Now *everything* is personal. We carry personal digital assistants and use personal protective equipment. We can hire personal trainers, personal assistants, and personal chefs.

Let's add another item to this growing list: the **personal health record (PHR)**. A PHR is a comprehensive, electronic or paper-based record of health information controlled by the individual, through which he or she can access, manage, and share confidential health information. With the proliferation of medical information in recent years, it's more important than ever for patients to maintain some control over it and to share responsibility with healthcare professionals for keeping the data up to date and accurate.

PHRs may be maintained by the patient or stored elsewhere, such as on the electronic health record (EHR), insurance carrier, or community health information exchange like Peacehealth or Healthbridge. Many employers, such as Wal-Mart and Intel, have arranged for their employees to have access to a PHR. The PHR is a means of keeping health information current, safe, and in a single location. The Centers for Medicare & Medicaid Services (CMS) support such initiatives as a way of reducing medical errors and cutting costs. In fact, CMS is pilot testing a PHR of its own in Utah, Arizona, and

BOX 8-1
Selected Web-Based Personal Health Records

HealthVault
www.healthvault.com
HealthVault is Microsoft's foray into the PHR arena. It is also in beta testing, although it appears to be farther along in the development process than the comparable Google product. HealthVault emphasizes health promotion tools, such as weight loss and blood pressure management. Microsoft has partnered with the manufacturers of several medical devices so that measurements can be downloaded from the devices and recorded directly into HealthVault.

My HealtheVet
www.myhealth.va.gov
This site, which is password protected after the patient registers, offers an online PHR tailored to the needs of veterans, including a medical library, podcasts, many health assessment and health promotion tools, and a place in which to record military medical history.

Web MD Health Manager
www.webmd.com/phr
Web MD offers a free PHR at this site. It includes A to Z disease information, drug guides, nutrition advice, and pregnancy and parenting information, as well as a template in which patients can store their health information. Some users may sign up for the Health Manager through their employers.

Careplan
www.careplan.co
Careplan is a web-based application that helps patient keep health information organized. Users can manage physician visits, medication lists, and contact information. Careplan also has tools for managing long-term illness like cancer, heart disease, and diabetes.

SynChart
www.synchart.com
SynChart is an online personal health record management system in which users can enroll themselves and up to seven family members for a small subscription fee (at time of print $9.95 per year). Elements of SynChart include emergency access, health report printing, medication summary, advance directives, living will, and immunizations.

South Carolina. Military veterans already have such a system (Box 8-1). In addition, the meaningful use program has cited patient portals as part of the stage 2 EHR usage requirements.

Recall from Chapter 1 that continuity of care encompasses the planning and coordination of care, which requires accessible healthcare information that can be shared with specialists and others during medical emergencies. Continuity of care also requires good communication between the patient and his or her providers and healthcare staff. A PHR improves continuity of care, particularly for those who move or switch providers frequently and for those who see multiple specialists, by consolidating health information. Like an EHR, it can also help the patient save time and money by keeping various specialists from ordering duplicate tests and procedures.

It's easy for patients to get lost in the myriad details of medication refills, appointment schedules, symptoms, diagnoses, and treatment instructions. Keeping a PHR may allow patients to get a bird's-eye view of their healthcare, perhaps spotting important trends or making connections between one symptom or condition and another. It's up to the provider to confirm the patient's hunch, of course, but gut instinct is important even in the analytic world of healthcare.

The Personal Health Record vs. The Medical Record

A PHR may sound an awful lot like an EHR. Both are a means of keeping health information up to date. Both offer some protection against loss of or damage to records that are stored elsewhere. And both aggregate data from physicians, hospitals, and allied health professionals into a single record.

The primary difference between a PHR and an EHR or a paper medical chart is who controls the data. Some observers have compared the concept of a PHR to that of a bank. Just as a bank account holder uses a PIN and ATM card for security, makes deposits, and writes checks, the PHR user accesses a password-protected account, **populates** the PHR with data, and decides to whom the data may be distributed and for what purposes. The patient can even specify that information from the PHR be disclosed only in emergency situations. Some systems, such as *My HealtheVet*, give users the option of printing emergency access information on a customized wallet card. Such information could be important in the event of a pandemic or a mass-casualty event such as a terrorist attack.

Because an individual is not a covered entity, the patient-controlled PHR is not subject to Health Insurance Portability and Accountability Act (HIPAA) privacy protection, nor does it necessarily constitute a legal document. However, if a provider, hospital, or other covered entity incorporates data from the PHR, the information becomes subject to HIPAA regulations. In addition, if a covered entity **hosts** a patient portal, it is required to provide the patient with a notice of privacy practice (NPP) that explains to the patient how the health information stored in it can be kept secure and confidential.

Researchers have found a closer connection between PHR systems and EHR systems than just their functionality, though (Trends and Applications 8-1). Physicians who have implemented EHR systems are aware of the benefits patient portals can offer the busy medical office, but many physicians are not convinced patient-controlled PHR systems can help the medical office yet. They are aware that patients use them and say that their patients' PHR systems were stored on some form of electronic media, such as a website or mobile application (app). However, the percentages of positive responses were low across the board. For example, only 7% of physician EHR adopters report that they actually use the information in their patient-controlled PHR systems.

TRENDS AND APPLICATIONS 8-1

The Personal Health Record: New Technology, New Questions

Relevance. Time-strapped practitioners worry that when patients share their PHR systems, providers will be expected to sift through heaps of clinically irrelevant information that patients have entered into their own records. Will providers be held legally responsible if, for instance, they did not read in paragraph 14 that Mrs. Verbosa was having occasional episodes of chest pain?

Communication. Many physicians are concerned that PHR systems or patient portals with messaging capabilities give the patient too much access to their providers. Studies have found, to the contrary, that patients tend to use email instead of calling, leaving practitioners with about the same workload as before.

Security. How can a patient's identity be authenticated once the PHR becomes interoperable with the EHR and other systems? What about the identities of caregivers authorized to view the patient's information? Patient portals will require user names and passwords, but it's up to the patient to keep that information secure.

Access. A question closely related to security is that of access. If a patient portal or gateway is used rather than a PHR, how much information should the practitioner give the patient, and which information should the patient be allowed to modify? Can patients be trusted to modify, if they wish, their allergy list, blood type, and other data for which accuracy is critical? So far, most patient portals are used to update demographics, schedule appointments, request medication refills, and pay bills.

Fragmentation. If a patient is using a PHR, the physician is unlikely to benefit from it if the patient chooses not to share the data. The problem is compounded if the data are not electronically compatible with the EHR used by the medical practice. Incompatible PHR systems

---

TRENDS AND APPLICATIONS 8-1—cont'd

make it more difficult to convey information to the provider and may serve to delay the implementation of nationwide interoperability standards for EHR systems and PHR systems.

   Upkeep. Maintenance is critical if a PHR is to remain useful to patients and their providers. Yet physicians and hospitals are still getting into the habit of sending copies of progress notes, lab reports, and similar documents to patients. When patients fail to receive or obtain copies of parts of their records, the PHR becomes incomplete and less useful, especially to emergency personnel and others not familiar with the patient's medical history. As upkeep is becoming easier, the meaningful use program requires eligible providers to make visit summaries available to a patient within 3 days of the encounter.

CRITICAL THINKING EXERCISE 8-1

How do you explain the connection between EHR adoption by the medical physician and PHR use by the patient? Does EHR use encourage patients to participate in their own healthcare? Or are proactive patients just more likely to patronize cutting-edge practices to begin with?

What Information Is Stored in a Personal Health Record?

The PHR should be a comprehensive collection of health information. Much like the EHR maintained by a medical office, the PHR should include information regarding patient demographics and past medical, family, and social history. It should provide ICE (in case of emergency) contact information for loved ones who should be notified if the patient is transported to a hospital and is unable to communicate.

   A PHR is also used to store information about a patient's allergies, current medications, and previous hospital and physician visits. In addition, a PHR may provide resources for managing patient illness and disease. For example, a patient with diabetes may include a link to the American Diabetes Association to obtain educational material related to the disease, or a recently discharged soldier might complete a screening tool to gauge his or her risk for posttraumatic stress disorder. Finally, patients sometimes store insurance information and claims payment history to keep a record of claims paid or denied. Box 8-2 lists information that a typical comprehensive PHR might contain.

BOX 8-2
What Does a PHR Contain?

Some PHR systems are created entirely by the patient, whereas others start with an online template at a web-hosting site. As a result, the information that a PHR might contain varies widely. It might consist of no more than a bare-bones summary of the individual's health history and emergency information. Other PHR systems comprise a detailed health record as well as a broad array of continually updated health promotion tools and information about diseases and conditions. Below are listed many of the items you might find in a comprehensive PHR:

Emergency Information
Patient's name, address, birth date, phone number, and Social Security number
Contact information for loved ones who should be notified if the patient is injured or killed or if the patient suddenly becomes ill
List of allergies to medications, foods, or other substances (latex, intravenous contrast solution, and so on)
Contact information for the patient's pharmacy
List of current medications, dosages, and prescribing physicians
Organ donor authorization

BOX 8-2—cont'd
What Does a PHR Contain?

Contact Information and Legal Documents
Health insurance information
Life insurance designation of beneficiary form
Contact information for physicians with whom the patient is established
Advance directive (including living will and medical power of attorney)
Contact information for dentists, therapists, or other healthcare providers

Family History
Health status or age and cause of death of first-degree relatives (mother, father, and siblings)
History of genetic or inherited diseases

Medical History
Chronologic list of surgical procedures and hospitalizations, including specific dates and treatment locations
List of acute illnesses and chronic diseases, including dates diagnosed, treatment received, providers' names, comments or notes to explain the event or condition, and correspondence with providers
List of accidents and injuries, including dates, treatment received, providers' names, and an explanation of the event and any residual problems linked to it, such as pain syndromes
History of exposure to toxic chemicals in the workplace or elsewhere
Documentation of physician visits
Results of laboratory, pathology, or imaging studies
Immunizations received, including dates and any adverse reactions
Vaccinations received, such as those for pneumonia and flu, and any adverse reactions

Social History
Occupation
Nutritional habits and physical activity regimen
Use of tobacco in any form
Use of alcohol or illegal drugs

Health Logs
Physical activity logs
Food journal
Blood glucose readings (especially for patients with diabetes or prediabetic conditions)
Blood pressure measurements
Cholesterol
Body temperature
Weight and body mass index (BMI)
Heart rate
Respiratory rate
Pain scale self-reports

Health Promotion Tools
Smoking cessation information and tools to track progress
Caregiver assistance, including lists of local resources
Advice for healthy eating, including logs to track food intake, weight, and physical activity
Self-care information about healthy sleep habits, including information on how to beat insomnia and when to visit a sleep clinic
Emergency preparedness resources, such as instructions for assembling a disaster preparedness kit and a first-aid kit
Mental health resources, such as information about stress and depression, numbers for suicide hotlines, and self-care advice for improving coping skills
Substance abuse resources, such as screening tools and links to information and help for those who may be abusing alcohol, prescription drugs, or illegal drugs

CRITICAL THINKING EXERCISE 8-2

Review the items in Box 8-2, then name three items not listed in the box that may be useful to store in a PHR.

In Chapter 3 we met Ellen, a 37-year-old, who has multiple sclerosis (MS). After a recent flare-up of her disease, Ellen had decided to take a more active role in her healthcare. She began requesting copies of her records from her physicians, including her neurologist, ophthalmologist, gastroenterologist, and general practitioner. In addition to receiving copies of these records, Ellen generated quite a bit of paperwork of her own, such as records requests, opt-out notices specifying to whom her health information can be disclosed, and a request for correction of erroneous information she discovered in her file.

Ellen was soon knee-high in a stack of operative summaries, authorization forms, and other documents, so she decided to organize it into a PHR. She wants her husband, Kent, who is her **caregiver** during her long periods of convalescence, to be able to find the information he needs if she isn't able to help him locate it, and she thinks a PHR will be a useful tool for doing so. In this chapter, we follow Ellen again as she creates and uses her new PHR.

CRITICAL THINKING EXERCISE 8-3

What type of person or patient is most likely to benefit from creating a PHR? What type of person or patient is most likely to create one? Are they the same?

Types of Personal Health Records

A patient like Ellen who has made the important decision to create a PHR must further decide whether to use a paper record, a stand-alone software program, or an online web-based PHR. Cost, portability, privacy, and other factors should be considered in making this decision.

Paper-Based Personal Health Records

Traditionally the PHR has been paper based. This method is inexpensive and secured as the patient's property. Paper-based PHR systems are generally organized into three-ring binders so that documents can easily be added or removed. Tabbed dividers, like those used in patient records kept in medical offices, can be used to organize and identify documents.

Of course, paper PHR systems have all the disadvantages of paper charts in a medical office. The chief drawback is the difficulty of sharing information. If the patient is ever crushed by a falling piano, say, or if he suddenly falls ill after eating tainted sushi, that tidy little three-ring binder sitting on a shelf in his home office won't do the emergency medical technicians much good. In addition, paper-based PHR systems require more work to maintain than patient portals. The user must remember to gather the data, and organize it in a timely manner. Patients that frequent a medical office or have a series of testing on a regular basis might find this overwhelming.

Personal Health Record Software

Patients who want to have their health information in electronic form but do not wish to store their private information online may decide to purchase a stand-alone software product. These programs allow the individual to create and save health information to a desktop or laptop computer. The files can also be made portable by saving them to a USB drive

Figure 8-1
USB drives, also called
thumb drives or *flash
drives.*

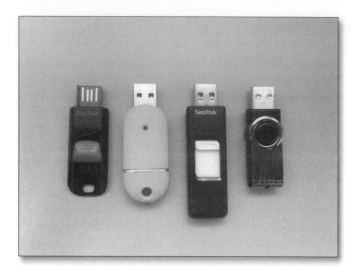

(also called a *thumb drive* or a *flash drive*), a small device that contains a digital memory chip on which electronic data can be stored and easily moved from one computer to another. A USB drive can be stored on a keychain and plugged in to most computers (Figure 8-1). Still, the files are not fully functional when the software is not available.

Online Personal Health Record

Many of us find it tough to imagine how we got by without computers to manage our lives. We use accounting software to compute our taxes, we check our credit card and bank balances on secure websites, we make dinner reservations and buy theater tickets online, and we even order stamps online when we need to send mail. Maintaining a web-based PHR, then, seems like a natural extension of the things we're already doing online.

Keeping a PHR in cyberspace means that it's accessible from any computer in the world that has an Internet connection. That's a big plus for patients like Ellen. She sometimes travels to a hospital in another state to one of her specialists, and she likes the idea of being able to pull up her PHR from her laptop. The hospital offers free **Wi-Fi**, so Ellen can even access her PHR from the lobby.

Many websites have been established at which patients can create free PHR systems and are even offered as apps installed in the patient's mobile devices for quick reference and use. Sites with advanced services and security generally charge a subscription fee. Another advantage of a web-based PHR is that it usually gives the patient easy access to a database of health information. Just as a medical assistant or provider using an EHR can quickly look up medication dosages, disease signs and symptoms, and evidence-based screening and treatment guidelines, the user of a web-based PHR can do so as well. Databases of information are not simply limited to medication either; apps like MyFitnessPal offer users nutritional information on just about every food you can think of to create food diaries and document physical activity.

Some health record sites are **patient portals,** tethered, physician-controlled gateways at which patients can not only maintain their health information but also request prescription refills, schedule appointments, pay bills, and send email to their healthcare providers. As part of stage 1 meaningful use requirements, providers must also provide access to problem lists, medication lists, and allergy records within 4 business days of the information being available to the provider. These sites, however, are not true PHR systems because although patients have some access to their records, the medical practice created the record and controls most of it. Perhaps it's more accurate to think of these kinds of records as patient-accessible (or at least partially accessible) EHR systems. Within such portals, the **patient-controlled health record** is the part of the site that contains data loaded by the patient and to which he or she alone may grant or deny access.

Careful research is a good idea before choosing a PHR. Dozens of choices are available, some of which are listed in Box 8-1. In addition, several Medicare Advantage or Part D drug plans offer PHR systems to their members. Ellen selected an online PHR with an extensive library of health information and a suite of health promotion tools. She also joined a free **social networking** site for people with MS. The sharing of personal health information through **online communities** is a great way for people like Ellen to feel connected with other individuals that share the same health concerns.

INNOVATIVE FEATURES OF PERSONAL HEALTH RECORDS

As you might imagine, PHR systems are capable of doing a great deal more than just storing personal health data and linking to medical and drug information. However, many of these features, some of which are described below, are fee-based add-ons that require a monthly or annual subscription. For some patients, especially those with chronic conditions and their caregivers, this may be money wisely spent. For others the money may be wasted because, like the clinical decision support (CDS) tools in an EHR, the features don't work if the patient doesn't use them.

Synchronization with Medical Devices

Some PHR systems are capable of linking directly to medical devices, such as scales, blood pressure cuffs, blood glucose meters for patients with diabetes, peak flow meters for patients with asthma, pedometers, and heart rate monitors. Using a USB connection—which is no more complicated than plugging in a lamp—measurements taken by the device can be downloaded directly into a tracking template on the PHR (Figure 8-2).

Figure 8-2
A spirometer with a USB connection capable of linking directly to a computer. (Courtesy of Welch Allyn.)

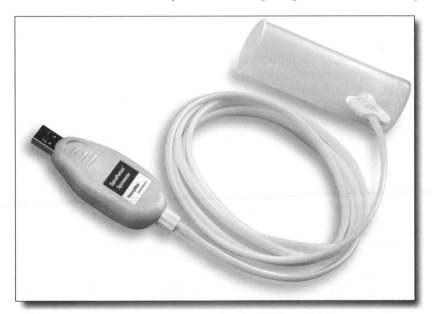

ICE Notification

Other applications allow the user to preselect which pieces of information from the PHR to make available to emergency personnel in the event of an accident of acute illness. The data can then be downloaded to a mobile device. Mobile apps like ICE, My Medical, and Emergency Contact are available for iPhone, Android, and iPad and are available for free to a few dollars to download. A wallet card can also be printed to give first responders instructions for accessing the information.

Ellen's PHR gave her the option of printing a summary of her essential medical information, along with login instructions for emergency personnel. She now carries the printed summary and a wallet card with her wherever she goes.

Drug Alerts

Just as a practitioner using an EHR receives a warning if he or she tries to prescribe a drug to which the patient is allergic or one that may cause an adverse reaction with another drug the patient takes, patients themselves can link their PHR systems to online software apps that will generate such alerts. The programs usually offer suggested alternatives to the medication being prescribed and send email alerts to the patient's provider. Some programs can even flag so-called drug-gene reactions if the patient has entered the results of genetic testing into the system. Mobile apps that focus on drug alerts such as Dosecase, Davis Mobile High Alert Drug, and MedCoach can help patients maintain and understand medication usage.

Limited Interoperability

Throughout this text we've discussed the concept of interoperability, the ability of separate systems to share information in compatible formats. Thus far, interoperability of PHR systems—with EHR systems, pharmacy systems, and so on—has proved elusive. Tang and colleagues warn that interoperability is critical if PHR systems are to avoid becoming "information islands" on which selected health data are isolated from the patient's main health record.

Parts of certain EHR systems are interoperable with certain external systems, though. For instance, urgent care clinics called MinuteClinic have entered into a strategic alliance with Microsoft's HealthVault to make all data from a patient's visit immediately downloadable to the patient's HealthVault PHR. If the patient goes to another urgent care clinic or chooses a different PHR, he or she loses this advantage (thus giving the patient an incentive to use both MinuteClinic and HealthVault).

Even if systems were interoperable, most medical practices have no electronic records system at all. Patients are asked to fill out tedious forms again and again. Some PHR systems, however, have a feature that allows patients to email their information to their physicians ahead of time. Practices that use paper charts can print the information and place the sheets right into the patient's chart. For a fee the information can be transferred to the actual forms used by a particular office. Patients can also scan documents, such as correspondence and **advance directive**s (including **living wills**), into their records. The physician can return information to the patient through the PHR as well, using secure email.

Direct-to-Consumer Laboratory Services

Our blood can reveal a lot about our health. In the past, a patient nearly always had to visit a physician to have a blood test ordered. Direct-to-consumer, web-based laboratory testing takes out the middleman. Let's say Chris, a 49-year-old man, is paying higher-than-average rates for life insurance because of his high cholesterol. He's been working out and watching his diet, using the PHR to track his progress, but Chris's insurance company will reassess his rates only once every 3 years. Chris wants to be sure his cholesterol has dropped before he requests a reassessment. Using a PHR that links him to a network physician who can submit the lab order and refer him to an approved facility, he can have the cholesterol test performed and have the results sent to his PHR account.

Telephone Consults

Worried parents, business travelers, and others with frequent need of a physician or temporary lack of access to one will appreciate the convenience of being able to share their PHR with a physician by telephone. There are fees attached to this service, but it may be less expensive and faster than paying for a visit to an urgent care center, assuming one is available. Patients should consider hidden charges, though, such as registration fees, that may be billed in addition to a monthly subscription fee and a flat-rate consultation fee.

Satellite and MP3 Technology

The satellite folks who can read our license plates from space continue to find creative uses for global positioning system (GPS) technology. Technology like FitBit allows users to monitor daily activities through a small bracelet worn daily. Susie Smith can map out a biking or walking route that's exactly 3.2 miles or whatever length she specifies. Or she can enter her current route to find out whether four laps around the dog park is really a whole mile. Then, drawing on the health goals and physical activity preferences she's outlined, the PHR can design a personal training session for her and combine it with her favorite Guns N' Roses tunes. When she's finished her workout, she can upload data from her heart rate monitor or pedometer into her PHR to find out and record how far she walked or rode, whether she reached her target heart rate, and how many calories she burned.

CRITICAL THINKING EXERCISE 8-4

Do you think a PHR or other health apps have the power to change an individual's health behavior? Why or why not?

Why Create a Personal Health Record?

In the introduction to this text and elsewhere, we reported that most physicians who adopt EHR systems say they'll never go back to paper. A similar point might be made about individuals who create PHR systems: They'll never go back to relying solely on their physicians to keep their health records for them.

Studies indicate that even though PHR systems haven't been around long, users already indicate a high rate of satisfaction with them. The PHR seems to have hopscotched over that bumpy period during which the bugs are worked out of a new technology. Perhaps that's because PHR systems are really just a novel application of many existing technologies. Little is known yet, say Tang and colleagues, about how people select PHR technology and integrate it into their lives. But the biggest implementation will come with physicians offering patient portals as a means to monitor health care.

For Ellen it made sense to create a PHR to help her keep track of information from multiple specialists and to gain more control over her healthcare decision making. She showed her PHR to Keira, one of her home health aides. Keira, whose physician had recently warned her that she showed signs of developing type 2 diabetes, decided to create a PHR for herself in order to monitor her weight, body mass index, heart rate, and physical activity. A Harris poll indicates that, like Keira and Ellen, more than half of Americans keep some sort of PHR. It stands to reason that the numbers will continue to grow.

Benefits to Individuals, Patients, and Caregivers

In this chapter we've tossed about the terms "individual," "consumer," "patient," and "PHR user" interchangeably, but a PHR isn't just for sick people. It's a powerful health promotion tool for those with no health problems, and it can help those with chronic conditions stay as healthy as possible by taking charge of their health. Keira, for example, discovered that keeping a PHR gave her additional motivation to stick to her fitness goals. She tracked her progress in her PHR and showed the encouraging results to her physician during her next visit.

Most PHR systems are more than just repositories of health information. They offer patients and caregivers the opportunity to do the following:

- Take an active role in a loved one's healthcare, particularly when those involved in care decisions—children of elderly parents, for instance—live in different parts of the country. (Remember, though, that the individual maintains control of the PHR if he or she is competent to do so. That means he or she must give permission to any family member who wants to access the information. Many PHR systems allow the patient to set up a separate password for others authorized to access the information in the record. A more permanent step is to grant **medical power of attorney** to a loved one and then file this information in the PHR.)

- Get a big-picture view that helps in planning and coordinating care.
- Learn about the diseases and conditions that affect them or their loved ones.
- Build friendships with and derive support from others who have the same condition.
- Lessen the likelihood that duplicate tests and procedures will be ordered.
- Monitor medications and potential drug interactions.
- Reduce the likelihood of medication errors and other medical errors.
- Follow physician self-care instructions for nutritional plans, postoperative self-care, and so on.
- Ensure that first responders can gain quick access to information in a medical emergency.
- Access data from anywhere (if an online PHR is chosen).
- Protect against unforeseen damage to or loss of information in the medical records maintained by their healthcare providers.
- Promote open communication among patients, providers, and staff.
- Improve continuity of care by consolidating health information from multiple specialists.
- Participate in researchers' tracking of population health trends.

In 2012, CNN posted a list of their top 10 mobile health apps. Here's who made the list:

1. **ZocDoc**—This is a free app that allows users to book physician appointments quickly. Patients simply enter their zip code and insurance information to click through available physicians, and book. (iPhone and Android)
2. **Zombies, Run!**—Zombies, Run! takes an unconventional approach to cardio, putting users in the shoes of zombie survivors outrunning the apocalypse. There are more than 30 missions and the high price ($7.99) hasn't dampened online appetite for the app. (iPhone, iPod Touch, iPad, Android, Windows)
3. **HealthTap**—This is a free healthcare Q&A station. Users can write and submit health care questions and get answers from real physicians. (iPhone and Android)
4. **MyFitnessPal**—MyFitnessPal is free and has a database with more than 2 million foods. It touts its fast and easy exercise and diet entry, allowing users to keep track of calorie burning and calorie intake on the go. (iPhone, iPod Touch, iPad, Android, BlackBerry, Windows)
5. **Stress Check**—This free app is both educational and diagnostic. It uses a one-step process—place an index finger on the camera lens of your phone—and then measures your stress level while supplying stress tips and tricks. (iPhone, iPod Touch, Android)
6. **Sleep Cycle**—This $0.99 alarm keeps track of users' sleeping patterns and then creates a 30-minute window around a preset alarm. Within that window, the app can then wake you from the lightest phase of sleep, which is the natural waking point. (iPhone, iPod Touch, iPod)
7. **Insight Timer**—With the sounds of Tibetan singing bowls as background noise, Insight Timer ($1.99) allows users to track their meditations, is customizable to individual meditation routines, and rewards achievement with insight "milestones." (iPhone, iPod Touch, iPad)
8. **Pocket Yoga**—A mobile guide to yoga, Pocket Yoga ($2.99) is customizable according to three different practices, difficulties, and durations, all created by Gaia Flow Yoga. Pose instructions come complete with voiceover, and users can swap out the default music for their own libraries. (iPhone, iPod Touch, iPad)
9. **Food on the Table**—This free recipe builder and shopping aid is rich with features. Users can search recipes, prefill their grocery lists, browse store discounts and

coupons, and even search for meal ideas with what's already on hand in the fridge. (iPhone, iPod Touch, iPad, Android)

10. **LifeKraze**—Users post their fitness goals in 160-character posts, plus photos or links on this free app. They're also given 300 points a day to reward others' accomplishments. Points can be redeemed for product discounts or donated to charity. The point system encourages people to exercise and urge others to do likewise. (iPhone, iPod Touch, iPad)

CRITICAL THINKING EXERCISE 8-5

Aside from security concerns, what reasons might there be for an individual not to create a PHR?

Benefits to Providers

Practitioners who view patients as partners in making healthcare decisions will appreciate the advantages a PHR offers. From a provider's perspective, PHR systems improve patients' compliance with instructions and medication regimens and generally improve patients' recall of health-related events. In addition, PHR systems give clinicians an alternative means of communicating with patients if secure email can be exchanged through the PHR.

CRITICAL THINKING EXERCISE 8-6

How do PHR systems benefit health insurance carriers?

STEPS IN CREATING THE PERSONAL HEALTH RECORD

Creating the PHR can seem like an overwhelming job, but patients should keep in mind that information does not need to be collected all at once. An easy way for patients to approach this task is to request copies of records during each of their next scheduled appointments with their healthcare providers and specialists. Users planning to implement web-based PHR systems should ask their physician how to log into the patient portal and obtain a username and password. Patients should also remember the payoff: Proper organization of the information will make it easy to locate when it's needed. There are three main steps users should follow in creating a PHR:

1. Decide which type of information to store in the PHR, and explore the methods of storing it.
2. Request copies of medical records from physicians' offices by signing records release forms, and be prepared to pay a fee for them. The patient may ask about the fee and time frame before making the request. It should only include the cost of copying supplies and labor and may take 60 to 90 days to complete. Inquire whether the office stores records in electronic format as an alternative to copying.
3. Begin collecting and organizing the health information. A three-ring binder may be the best way initially to organize the documents. Tabbed, color-coded dividers help separate the different types of information. Once the health information has been organized, it can be transferred to another method of storage, such as a web page or software application, according to the patient's preference. Some health forms may be downloaded from free PHR sites to aid the organization of patient health information. Figure 8-3 shows a sample of one such form. To download the complete form, visit www.myphr.com.

Figure 8-3 Sample health forms that may be used in a PHR. (From www.myPHR.com; © 2006 by the American Health Information Management Association. All rights reserved.)

Health Information Form *for Adults*

AHIMA
American Health Information Management Association®

A. IDENTIFICATION

Name (Last) (First) (Middle)

Maiden Name

Primary Address

City	State	Zip Code	Country

Alternate Address

City	State	Zip Code	Country

Home Phone	Work Phone
Cell Phone	E-mail Address

Date of Birth	☐ Male	☐ Female

Height	Weight	Eye Color	Hair Color

Ethnicity/Race	Birthmarks/Scars

Blood / RH Type	Special Conditions	Marital Status

Occupation

Company Name

Address

City	State	Zip Code	Country

Phone Number	Languages Spoken—Primary and Secondary
Primary Health Insurance Carrier	Policy Number
Secondary Health Insurance Carrier	Policy Number

B. EMERGENCY CONTACTS

In Case of Emergency, Notify: Primary Contact

Name (Last) (First) (Middle)

Relationship

Address

City	State	Zip Code	Country

Home Phone	Work Phone
Cell Phone	E-mail Address

In Case of Emergency, Notify: Secondary Contact

Name (Last) (First) (Middle)

Relationship

Address

City	State	Zip Code	Country

Home Phone	Work Phone
Cell Phone	E-mail Address

In Case of Emergency, Notify: Medical Contact

Physician (Indicate Specialty)

Phone

Dentist	Phone
Pharmacy	Phone

Figure 8-3, cont'd Sample health forms that may be used in a PHR.

Health Information Form *for Adults*

AHIMA
American Health Information
Management Association®

Page No.

C. HEALTHCARE PROVIDERS

Healthcare Provider Speciality	Primary Care Physician ☐ Yes ☐ No	Phone	Emergency Phone No. (after hours)
Name		E-mail Address	
Group or Association		Fax	
Address		Web Address/URL	
City	State	Zip Code	Country		

Healthcare Provider Speciality	Primary Care Physician ☐ Yes ☐ No	Phone	Emergency Phone No. (after hours)
Name		E-mail Address	
Group or Association		Fax	
Address		Web Address/URL	
City	State	Zip Code	Country		

Healthcare Provider Speciality	Primary Care Physician ☐ Yes ☐ No	Phone	Emergency Phone No. (after hours)
Name		E-mail Address	
Group or Association		Fax	
Address		Web Address/URL	
City	State	Zip Code	Country		

Healthcare Provider Speciality	Primary Care Physician ☐ Yes ☐ No	Phone	Emergency Phone No. (after hours)
Name		E-mail Address	
Group or Association		Fax	
Address		Web Address/URL	
City	State	Zip Code	Country		

MAINTAINING THE PERSONAL HEALTH RECORD

Although the patient may spend a great deal of time up front to populate and organize the PHR, that time will be wasted if maintenance isn't a top priority. A dated PHR is useless. Smolij and Dun, who studied various models of managing health information, believe that patients' lack of diligence in updating the PHR and their questionable judgment about what to include in it make the PHR "highly unreliable and its validity and value questionable." Perhaps, though, this statement says more about some physicians' paternal attitude toward patients as a barrier to PHR use than it does about the value of the PHR.

CRITICAL THINKING EXERCISE 8-7

One might argue that any patient who takes the initiative to create a PHR and spends at least several hours populating it probably has a good grasp of what information is important to include and what may safely be excluded. Do you agree with this line of reasoning? Why or why not?

Each time patients are seen by a healthcare provider, they may need to sign a specific authorization for the medical office to release their records. (Some PHR systems offer, for a fee, conversion of a patient's existing medical records and health-related documents into a PHR by a trained nurse-abstractor. The patient can purchase a monthly subscription to have new information added as it is generated, ensuring that the record stays up to date.) Ellen used the records release offered as a free download in her PHR. Each time she had an appointment with a physician, she simply opened the file and changed the date on the request before printing and signing it. Then she took the request with her to the visit.

Patients should be sure to log their weight, any immunizations or vaccinations given, laboratory results, results of imaging studies (for instance, colon and breast cancer screenings), vital signs, medication changes, and the findings of physical examinations. The information entered should always be accompanied by a date. Many PHR systems provide templates in which such information can be logged and easily retrieved.

CHAPTER SUMMARY

- The PHR is a comprehensive collection of patient health information maintained in one central location and controlled by the patient. A PHR and an EHR both keep health information current, offer some insurance against damage to records stored elsewhere, and consolidate data from physicians, hospitals, and allied health professionals into a single record. The primary difference between a PHR and an EHR or a paper medical chart is who controls the information in the record. Because an individual is not a covered entity, the PHR is not subject to HIPAA privacy protection and does not necessarily constitute a legal document, although it may be accepted as evidence in some court cases. Information about medication allergies, a list of current medications, immunization records, loved ones' contact information, organ donor and living will instructions, and a brief medical, social, and family history are essential information in any PHR. Detailed documents supporting this information, such as scans of correspondence and full lab results, help to confirm accuracy but are not essential. Health promotion tools, such as smoking cessation logs, are other optional additions to the PHR.
- Traditionally the PHR has been a paper-based document kept in a simple three-ring binder. This method is inexpensive, easy to maintain, and secure. Its chief drawback is the difficulty of sharing information. Patients who want to have their health information in an electronic format but do not wish to store their private information

online may decide to purchase a stand-alone software product. The files, but not the full functionality of the PHR, can be made portable by saving them to a USB drive. Creating a PHR online means the patient's health record is accessible from any computer in the world that has an Internet connection and offers the bonus of easy access to health information. Although a basic web-based PHR may be free, those with advanced services and security generally charge a subscription fee.

- Using its advanced health promotion features, a patient can synchronize the PHR with a variety of medical devices, such as blood pressure cuffs and heart rate monitors. Doing so allows, for example, patients with hypertension to monitor their blood pressure and fitness over time, easily tracking the data in their EHR, and, if they choose, sharing it with their physician.

- Interoperability of PHR systems with EHR systems and other systems, such as hospital and pharmacy networks, is critical if PHR systems are to become a viable means of sharing patients' health data, rather than isolating it.

- Direct-to-consumer laboratory services can allow patients to control who sees the results of their blood tests.

- Having a PHR can help individuals who create it get a big-picture view of their healthcare, learn about diseases and conditions, build relationships with others who have the same condition, save money on duplicate tests and procedures, communicate openly with healthcare personnel, take an active role in a loved one's healthcare, monitor medications, reduce the likelihood of medication errors and interactions, follow self-care instructions, give first responders quick access to information in a medical emergency, access data from anywhere, protect against unforeseen loss of information, improve continuity of care, and participate in researchers' tracking of population health trends. From a provider's perspective, PHR systems do all of the above as well as improve patients' compliance with instructions and medication regimens, improve patients' recall of health-related events, and give the clinician an alternative means of communicating with patients.

- Selecting a storage device, obtaining medical records, submitting records release forms, and organizing health information are all important steps in establishing a PHR.

- The time spent initially populating and organizing a PHR will be wasted if patients don't make maintenance a top priority. To do so, they must collect copies of progress notes, prescriptions, and other documents on each visit to a healthcare provider.

CHAPTER REVIEW ACTIVITIES

Key Terms Review

Match the term in column A to the definition in column B.

1. Medical power of attorney
2. Advance directive
3. Host site
4. Caregiver
5. Populate
6. Patient portal
7. Personal health record
8. Living will
9. Personally controlled health record
10. Wi-Fi
11. Social networking

a. The *part* of an advanced directive naming a trusted person to make medical decisions on the patient's behalf should he or she become unable to make such decisions independently

b. Legal document outlining a person's wishes regarding which treatments should be administered or withheld if the person becomes incapacitated

c. To complete a template or create a record by providing the missing information for a set of predetermined fields

d. Provides information and services, such as secure email, access to an online appointment book, and limited access to patient records

e. Secure, comprehensive record of health information that is controlled by the individual

f. A person who provides physical care and emotional support to a person who is ill, disabled, or dependent

g. The *part* of an advance directive that specifies which life-sustaining treatments should be administered or withheld if the person becomes incapacitated

h. The point at which a website originates or resides

i. The practice of using online communities to expand one's contacts and exchange content

j. A means of connecting wirelessly to the Internet using a local area network or router

k. The portion of a patient portal to which the patient has access and may grant or deny access

True/False

Indicate whether the statement is true or false.

1. _____ A PHR may be paper based or electronic.

2. _____ The primary difference between a PHR and an EHR or a paper medical chart is its storage location.

3. _____ The PHR is a legal health record with the same legal standing as an EHR under HIPAA.

4. _____ A list of current allergies and medications should be included in the PHR.

5. _____ Patients may use the PHR to share health information with caregivers in order to better understand their medical treatments and manage disease.

6. _____ The information in stand-alone PHR systems created with software programs is not portable into other systems.

7. _____ An online PHR is accessible from any computer in the world that has an Internet connection.

8. _____ All PHR systems require membership and setup fees in addition to purchase of a monthly subscription.

9. _____ Some PHR systems integrate satellite technology to help users plan biking or walking routes.

10. _____ Patients portals are more present than ever in medical offices because of the meaningful use requirement.

Workplace Applications

1. Visit www.webmd/phr.com and register for a free PHR. What type of health assessments are used in this free service? Describe the advantages and disadvantages of using this site to maintain a patient PHR.

2. Using a search engine, identify four different websites and apps (other than those given in this chapter) for creating and maintaining a PHR and other health-related information. What are the strengths and weaknesses of each site? What kinds of resources and tools are provided to users? What security measures are taken to ensure confidentiality? Are the sites free, or do they have charges associated with them?

3. Your office is implementing a patient portal to their EHR. This transition will occur next month and patients will be given login information at regular office visits. There will be all staff training for the patient portal on next Tuesday from 4 to 5 PM in the meeting room. Use SimChart for the Medical Office (SCMO) to set the training in the Calendar. Then use the email Correspondence tool to create an Office Memo informing staff of this training and agenda.

4. Mora Siever (01/24/1964) is in the process of collecting data for her PHR. She comes to the office today to complete a patient records access request form to review the contents of her health record as part of this goal. She is interested in accessing all progress notes, immunizations, and radiology and laboratory reports from 2005 to the present for the creation of her PHR.

EHR in Review

1. Ken Thomas (10/25/1961) had a form completed by Dr. Walden for a life insurance policy. The fee for form completion is $20.00. Update the patient's ledger to reflect this charge.

2. The following office expenses were incurred during the month of November. Complete the Petty Cash journal. The amount of Petty Cash on hand at the start of the month is $200.00. Enter "date reconciled" as today. Once the posting is complete, what is the amount of Petty Cash on Hand? (Subtract starting amount to expenses)

DATE	DESCRIPTION	EXPENSE
11/02/20XX	Postage	21.80
11/08/20XX	Shuttle to hospital	8.00
11/16/20XX	Facial tissue	35.00
11/21/20XX	Napkins and plates for Thanksgiving luncheon	27.08

3. Jean Burke, NP, has ordered an electrolyte panel for Tai Yan (04/07/1956) for chronic kidney disease (CKD). Create a lab requisition for the patient using Form Repository and update the patient's Problem list to include CKD. (You may need to create an encounter to document the Problem List if one does not already exist.)

4. Norma Washington (08/01/1944) calls the office today. She cannot remember when her next appointment is scheduled. Use the Calendar search to located Norma's next appointment.

BIBLIOGRAPHY

Ball, M. J., & Gold, J. (2006). Banking on health: Personal records and information exchange. *Journal of Healthcare Information Management*, 20(2), 78–81.

Fuji, K. T., Galt, K. A., & Serocca, A. B. (2008). Personal health record use by patients as perceived by ambulatory care physicians in Nebraska and South Dakota: A cross-sectional study. *Perspectives in Health Information Management*, 5, 15.

Halamka, J. D., Mandl, K. D., & Tang, P. C. (2008). Early experiences with personal health records. *Journal of the American Medical Informatics Association*, 15(1), 1–7.

Harris Interactive. (2004). Two in five adults keep personal or family health records and almost everybody thinks this is a good idea. *Harris Interactive Health Care News*, 13(4), 1–5. Available at: www.harrisinteractive.com/news/newsletters/healthnews/HI_HealthCareNews2004Vol4_Iss13.pdf. Accessed 01.03.09.

Tang, P. C., Ash, J. S., Bates, D. W., et al. (2006). Personal health records: Definitions, benefits, and strategies for overcoming barriers to adoption. *Journal of the American Medical Informatics Association*, 13, 121–126.

Taylor, H. (2008). Number of "cyberchondriacs"—adults going online for health information—has plateaued or declined. *Harris Interactive Healthcare News*, 8(8). Available at: www.harrisinteractive.com/news/newsletters/healthnews/HI_HealthCareNews2008Vol8_Iss8.pdf. Accessed 01.03.09.

Smolij, K., & Dun, K. (2006). Patient health information management: searching for the right model. *Perspectives in Health Information Management*, 3, 10.

Glossary

abuse Unintentional deception in which a provider inappropriately bills for services that are not medically necessary, do not meet current standards of care, or are not medically sound.

account ledger An accounting billing document that lists services provided, copayments made by the patient, reimbursement received from the patient's insurance company, and outstanding amount owed.

active patient An established patient who has seen the provider, or another provider in the billing group within the past 3 years.

acute condition An illness or injury that is episodic (e.g., a seizure), has a sudden onset (such as a broken bone), is of limited duration (e.g., bronchitis), and generally responds well to prompt medical attention.

advance directive A binding legal document prepared and signed by a competent individual outlining the person's wishes should the person become incapacitated. Components of an advance directive may include a medical power of attorney and a living will.

adverse action A decision by an insurance company, such as a health or disability insurer, to deny or terminate insurance or to increase rates, usually based on information obtained from a consumer reporting agency.

anonymity The patient's right, which exists to varying degrees, to have private health data collected in a way that can never be linked or traced back to him or her.

anthropometric measurements Measurements of height, weight, and size used to compare the relative proportions of the human body in health and illness.

application service provider A company that provides on-line access to a software application; requires a licensing agreement with the end-user. Application service provider arrangements allow the end-user to access software over the Internet and can be a less expensive alternative to purchasing a copy of the software and installing it on the user's local (on-site) server.

applications software (usually referred to simply as "application") A program or suite of programs with word processing, graphics, database, spreadsheet, or other capabilities that is used to accomplish work-related tasks for the user.

audit A review of employee activity within the EHR system, including an examination of which files were accessed or modified, as well as when and why.

audit trail A record that traces a user's electronic footsteps by recording activity and transactions, including unsuccessful attempts to view unauthorized screens, within the EHR system.

authentication The process of determining whether the person attempting to access a given network or EHR system is authorized to do so. User authentication can include password entry or use of biometric data (such as a digital fingerprint or voice signature) or a smart card (a data-laden microchip).

authorization A document giving a covered entity permission to use protected health information for specified purposes other than treatment, payment, or healthcare operations or to disclose protected health information to a third party specified by the patient.

button An element of the user interface on which the user can click to execute a command, such as confirm, cancel, or exit.

caregiver A person responsible for providing physical care and emotional support, usually in a home-care setting, to a person who is ill, disabled, or dependent.

Certification Commission for Healthcare Information Technology (CCHIT) A recognized certification body for EHRs and their networks. The CCHIT is an independent, voluntary, private-sector initiative whose goal is to accelerate the adoption of health information technology.

check box A specialized type of button that toggles on (checked) and off (unchecked). Check boxes are often used when more than one response might be appropriate (as in "Check all that apply"), but sometimes they should be interpreted to mean yes or no (as in a check box next to the caption "OK to mail?").

chief complaint (CC or cc) A brief statement noted on each visit, usually in the patient's own words, of the problem, condition, or symptoms that prompted the patient to seek medical care.

chronic condition An illness that persists for a prolonged period (typically 3 months or longer) and requires periodic follow-up with a healthcare provider, regardless of whether the condition has a sudden or gradual onset.

client-server model An architecture in which a powerful central computer serves a network of connected PCs or other workstations, called clients. The interface that allows the client and server to communicate (Windows or Linux, for example) resides on the client's computer. The software application and stored files (patients' EHRs) reside on the server, which shares them when it receives a request from the client.

clinical decision support (CDS) A set of patient-centered tools embedded within EHR software that can be used to improve patient safety, ensure that care conforms to published protocol for specific conditions, and reduce duplicate or unnecessary care and its associated costs.

cloning Copying and pasting notes from a patient's previous visit into the current progress note (also called "carrying forward") or pasting notes from one patient's record into the record of a patient with a similar diagnosis and presentation.

closed patient record The record of a patient who has not been seen by the provider, or any other provider in the billing group in 3 or more years.

coding variance Medical coding mistakes caused by computer error or by various kinds of human error, from simple carelessness to incorrect application of coding guidelines and procedures.

coinsurance A percentage of the total amount of the bill that is applied after the deductible.

compliance plan A written set of office policies and procedures intended to ensure compliance with laws regulating billing, coding, and third-party reimbursement.

computerized physician order entry (CPOE) An EHR function that allows a physician or other prescriber to order medications and tests using an automated format; CPOE can reduce prescribing errors, delays, and duplication and simplify inventory and billing processes.

confidentiality The patient's right and expectation that individually identifiable health information will be kept private and not disclosed without the patient's permission. Confidentiality is limited or protected by law to varying degrees.

consent Permission given to a covered entity for uses and disclosures of protected health information for treatment, payment, and health care operations.

consultation According to the Centers for Medicare & Medicaid Services (CMS), a request for advice from a doctor or other qualified practitioner whose opinion or advice regarding the evaluation or management of a specific problem is requested by another doctor.

consumer reporting agency An agency regulated by the Federal Trade Commission (FTC) under the Fair Credit Reporting Act (FCRA) that sells or cooperatively exchanges consumer information and history in areas such as credit and healthcare.

context specific Generated to help the user in a specific context or to carry out a particular task; refers to a feature or function of a software application, such as a context-specific help menu or a context-specific toolbar.

continuity of care A key aspect of quality that encompasses planning and coordination of care, communication among members of the healthcare team, and accessibility and transportability of information.

controlled vocabulary A standardized list of preferred terms for medical diagnoses, findings, procedures, services, and treatments, along with machine-readable numeric codes that identify them. Examples include ICD diagnosis codes, CPT procedure codes, and NDC prescriptions codes.

copayment A fixed, out-of-pocket expense for covered services specified by the patient's healthcare plan and due at the time the services are rendered.

covered entities Healthcare providers, health plans, and healthcare clearinghouses that transmit claims electronically. As part of covered entities, business associates are those who are contracted by covered entities to perform specific duties and have a corresponding contract detailing their responsibilities.

CPT-4 *Current Procedural Terminology*, fourth edition. A comprehensive set of medical codes and corresponding labels that describes procedures, treatments, and services for the purpose of determining reimbursement rates.

data capture The process of indirectly entering data into a system by recording (capturing) it electronically and converting it to machine-readable form. Examples of data capture methods include bar coding, voice recognition software, and structured templates.

day sheet A register for daily business transactions; also called a day journal.

default A preselected value or setting that will be used unless the user specifies a substitute by overriding the preselected choice.

disclosure Giving access to, releasing, or transferring information to a person or entity not legally or ethically authorized to use or have knowledge of it.

documentation The process of recording data about a patient's health history and status, including clinical observations and progress notes, diagnoses of illnesses and injuries, plans of care, patient education and self-care instructions given, vital signs taken, physical assessment findings, laboratory and imaging test results, medical treatments prescribed or administered, surgeries performed, and outcomes; the term can also refer to the chronologic record that results from such data entry.

double-booking Giving two or more patients the same appointment slot with the same provider.

electronic data interchange (EDI) An information exchange technology that facilitates the rapid, accurate transfer of encrypted data in a standardized, mutually agreed-upon format.

electronic health record (EHR) A computerized patient health record that allows the electronic management of a patient's health information by multiple healthcare providers and stores the patient's contact information, legal documents, demographic data, and administrative information; the term can also refer more broadly to a system that manages such records.

electronic transcription Data entry into the EHR using handwriting recognition, voice recognition, electronic sentence building, scanning, and other means.

encounter a documented interaction or visit between a patient and health care provider.

encounter form A form generated to reflect the services and charges for a patient visit. It includes patient information, account balance, and follow-up instructions.

encryption technology A system that keeps data secure by converting it to an unreadable code during transmission and then unencrypting the information when it reaches the recipient.

ethics Rules and standards of conduct that govern professional behavior and arise from our shared understanding of morality.

e-visit An evaluation and management service provided by a doctor or other qualified health professional to an established patient using a web-based or similar electronic-based communication network for a single patient encounter that occurs over safe, secure, online communication systems.

fax machine A device capable of encoding documents and sending them over a telephone line; a secure fax sends fax transmissions via secure email, eliminating many of a fax's security risks.

field Space allocated on a form for specific numeric or text data.

fraud Presenting (or causing to be presented) claims for services that an individual or entity knows or should know to be false.

go live   To become operational; the point at which the offline practice mode ends and real-world, online use begins. Often used in the phrase "go-live date."

guarantor   The person who bears ultimate financial responsibility for a patient's account; usually the guarantor is the patient, but the guarantor for a minor or a person of decreased mental capacity may be a parent, trustee, or legal guardian.

high-alert medication   A medication that poses a heightened risk of injury or death when administered improperly.

HIPAA 5010   The standard claim format used by a noninstitutional provider or supplier to submit a claim electronically to Medicare and most other insurance carriers for covered services.

history of the present illness (HPI)   Details about the duration, time, location, severity, context, associated signs and symptoms, quality, and modifying factors related to the patient's illness.

host   A server that provides data transfer, storage space, and other services to users at remote locations; a host has a unique domain name and is, in effect, the point at which a website originates.

hybrid   A medical office in which health records are stored and accessed in various formats—paper charts, EHRs, and perhaps microfilm, microfiche, or other media.

ICD-10-CM   International Classification of Diseases, Tenth Revision, with Clinical Modification. A coding system used to describe inpatient and outpatient diagnoses.

individually identifiable health information (IIHI)   Health information that clearly identifies an individual patient or could reasonably be used to identify the patient; see *protected health information (PHI)*.

interoperability   The ability of separate EHR systems to share information in compatible formats.

laws   Formal, enforceable rules and policies based on community standards of conduct.

legacy   A functional EHR system slated to be replaced with newer software.

letter templates   Standardized, preconstructed documents that address specific topics but can be tailored to individual recipients.

living will   The part of an advance directive that specifies which life-sustaining treatments (for example, mechanical ventilation and tube feeding) should be administered or withheld if the person becomes incapacitated.

macro   A single, user-defined computer instruction that, when processed, executes a complex series of commands.

medical coding   The process of assigning standard numeric or alphanumeric codes to diagnoses, procedures, and treatments for research, disease tracking, and reimbursement purposes.

medical identity theft   The unauthorized use of someone else's personal information to obtain medical services or submit fraudulent medical insurance claims for reimbursement.

medical power of attorney (also called durable power of attorney for healthcare or healthcare proxy)   The part of an advance directive naming a trusted person to make medical decisions on the patient's behalf should he or she become unable to make such decisions independently.

medication reconciliation   The process of comparing the medication list in the patient's EHR with the patient's self-report of the medications he or she has been taking.

minimum necessary standard   A key provision of the HIPAA Privacy Rule requiring that disclosures include no more than the minimum necessary amount of information to accomplish a given purpose.

no-show   A patient who makes an appointment and neither shows up nor calls to cancel; the term also refers to the appointment itself (a "no-show appointment").

objective   Readily seen, perceived, or measured by the clinician, not only by the patient.

off-label indication   A use for a prescription drug other than that for which the U.S. Food and Drug Administration (FDA) has approved it.

online community   A virtual meeting space where like-minded people with common interests or concerns interact and build relationships using real-time chat rooms, asynchronous threaded discussions, discussion groups, social media, news groups, web conferencing, and other technologies.

organizational culture   The shared set of values, beliefs, and assumptions that governs the perceptions and interactions of the organization's members and guides their behavior and decision making.

password   A sequence of characters and sometimes spaces used to prevent unauthorized access to or disclosure of patient information contained in secure electronic files.

patient flow   The efficient movement of patients through the medical office as a product of accurately estimated patient volume, a consistent provider pace, and efficient scheduling practices; the term generally refers to the overall flow of patients but can refer to the path of an individual patient.

patient information form   A form used to gather data about the patient, including basic demographics, medical insurance data and emergency contact.

patient portal   A website that serves as an information transfer hub between patient and physician and provides information and services, such as secure email, search capabilities, access to an online appointment book, and limited access to patient records.

patient-controlled health record   The portion of a patient portal that contains data loaded by the patient and to which he or she alone may grant or deny access.

pay for performance (P4P)   An outcomes-based payment model that offers providers financial incentives for meeting specific standards and electronically documenting compliance with them; punitive measures may be applied to providers who fail to comply.

personal health record (PHR)   A secure, comprehensive record of health information that is controlled by the individual, creating a confidential electronic or paper-based file that is easy to access, manage, and share.

PFSH   An abbreviation for past (medical), family, and social history.

populate   To complete a template or create a record by filling in a set of predetermined fields with information ranging from demographic data to values and measurements (for example, vital signs) to entire documents (such as correspondence and operative reports).

postural blood pressure (posturals) Blood pressure readings taken in different positions: recumbent, sitting, or standing.

practice management software Software used in a medical office to accomplish administrative (nonclinical) tasks, including entry of patient demographics, record-keeping for insurance and other billing transactions, appointment scheduling, and advanced accounting functions.

preimplementation process The process of training the staff and gathering the resources necessary to implement a conversion from a paper-based or legacy EHR to a new EHR system; the preparation phase that occurs before the go-live date.

privacy The patient's freedom to determine when, how much, and under what circumstances his or her medical information may be disclosed.

protected health information (PHI) Individually identifiable health information that is stored, maintained, or transmitted electronically; in practice, however, this term is often used interchangeably with the term IIHI, regardless of what form the information takes.

purging The process of separating inactive patient health records from active ones.

radio button A specialized type of button on a software interface that toggles on (round button visible) and off (blank circle). Radio buttons tell the user that only one response is appropriate, because two radio buttons can't be depressed at the same time.

records management The systematic control of patient records, from creation through maintenance and storage.

referral The recommendation of a patient to another healthcare provider for more specialized treatment, testing, or consultation; referrals are usually given by general practitioners to specialist doctors.

refresh To reload the page or update it with current data.

request for proposal A formal written request sent to a shortlist of software vendors outlining the practice's needs, resources, time frame, and budget, and requesting specific information about customer support, software features and proposed platform, tentative preimplementation plan, and estimated costs.

retention period The amount of time patient records must, by law, be maintained by the medical office.

review of systems (ROS) An organized inventory of each organ system, completed as part of the initial patient interview to pinpoint any unusual findings in the patient's history.

safeguards Measures taken to prevent interference with computer network operations and to avert security breaches involving the unauthorized use, disclosure, modification, erasure, or destruction of protected health information; these measures are specified by the HIPAA Security Rule, which applies only to data in electronic form.

screensaver A program that displays moving text or images on the screen if input (such as a keystroke) is not received for a given time period.

secondary use A use of health information that is not directly related to patient care. Such uses include statistical analysis; research, quality, and safety assurance processes; public health monitoring; payment; provider certification or accreditation; and marketing and other business activities.

secure email An email system capable of transmitting an encrypted message and storing it in coded format until it is retrieved by the recipient via a secure web link.

show rate The percentage of patients in a practice who arrive for appointments as scheduled or call in advance to cancel or reschedule.

social networking The practice of using online communities to expand one's social or business contacts and exchange content, such as images and instant messages; the term also refers to the broader phenomenon of this practice, which has created virtual communities with millions of members.

speech recognition A technology that converts speech into text.

structured data entry Use of mouse clicks, touch-screen commands, or simple keystroke combinations to enter data that conform to a controlled vocabulary; structured data entry helps practitioners input a large amount of information efficiently and is appropriate for describing typical signs, symptoms, and other straightforward clinical facts and findings.

subjective Perceived only by the patient and not evident to or measurable by the clinician.

telephone etiquette A polite, helpful response and respectful manner toward callers that shows patients they are cared for and valued.

template Predefined, customizable forms that facilitate structured data collection by offering the clinician a set of menus, check boxes, and other tools with which to enter data into progress notes, letters, and other EHR documents.

third-party payer An individual or entity other than the patient (the first party) or the provider (the second party) that is financially responsible for a portion of the patient's healthcare bills.

unstructured data entry Free data entry (as opposed to structured data entry using a controlled vocabulary) using direct keying, dictation, or transcription; unstructured data entry is needed to describe nuanced patient presentations and unique individual health histories.

views Different ways of displaying the same or similar information on a computer screen, usually with an increasing or decreasing level of detail (for example, looking at an electronic calendar in daily, weekly, and monthly views).

virtual private network A pathway that allows encrypted data to travel securely through an Internet connection to its destination, where it is unencrypted.

Wi-Fi (short for Wireless Fidelity, a technologic certification body) A means of connecting wirelessly to the Internet using a local area network or router.

workflow A set of related tasks necessary to complete a step in a business process.

Index

Page numbers followed by *b*, *t*, and *f* indicate boxes, tables, and figures, respectively.